How to beat fatigue

How
to
beat
fatigue

Linda Pembrook

Introduction by Donald T. Fredrickson, M.D.

Doubleday & Company, Inc.
Garden City, New York

1975

Some of the material in "Getting Control of Time" is reprinted from the book *How to Get Control of Your Time and Your Life* by Alan Lakein, published by Peter H. Wyden, Publishers, a division of David McKay Co., Inc. Copyright © 1973 by Alan Lakein. Used with permission.

Library of Congress Cataloging in Publication Data

Pembrook, Linda.
    How to beat fatigue.

    Includes bibliographies.
    1. Fatigue. 2. Hygiene. 3. Fatigue, Mental.
4. Stress (Psychology) I. Title. [DNLM: 1. Fa-
tigue—Popular works. WB146 P396h]
RA776.5.P4   612'.04
ISBN 0-385-01928-9
Library of Congress Catalog Card Number 74–25120

To

Duke Yates and Al Roller

CONTENTS

INTRODUCTION   ix

PART ONE
Physical fatigue

Chapter 1   Defining Fatigue   7
Chapter 2   Getting Control of Time   17
Chapter 3   How Much Sleep Is Enough?   27
Chapter 4   Noise Is Tiring   43
Chapter 5   Exercise Keeps You Young   49
Chapter 6   You Are What You Eat   65
Chapter 7   Drugs and Alcohol: Tired People Beware   87
Chapter 8   The State of Your Health   105

PART TWO
Emotional fatigue

Chapter 9   The Tired Housewife   121
Chapter 10   Sexual Fatigue: "Too Tired" Is No Excuse   139
Chapter 11   The Awesome Influence of Stress   145
Chapter 12   How Anxieties Wear You Out   163
Chapter 13   Fatigue as Masked Depression   181
Chapter 14   Fighting Boredom   197
Chapter 15   Conclusion   217

INTRODUCTION

The past three decades have seen remarkable changes in the practice of medicine. Much of this has resulted from an explosion in scientific knowledge and technique. During the early years of this century, pneumonia, meningitis, dysentery, tuberculosis, and other infectious diseases were the principal causes of disability and death. With the introduction of antibiotics in the late 1930s—first the sulfa drugs, then penicillin, and finally the broad-spectrum antibiotics—we literally revolutionized medical practice and overnight dramatically changed the course of human illnesses that had plagued mankind for centuries. With a cure for infectious diseases at hand, many thought we would enter a new era of almost unlimited physical health and well-being. But the millennium did not arrive, for in solving one problem we unmasked another. We made it possible for people to live longer and, thereby, to become heir to a new set of ailments—heart disease, emphysema, cancer, arthritis—the chronic debilitating diseases.

At the same time something else was happening that was to influence patterns of health and disease in the developed countries. We moved from an agricultural to an industrialized way of life with the rapid growth of mass transportation and instant communication systems and this worked profound changes in the nature of man's relationship to the world around him. In part this was characterized by a general loosening of traditional beliefs and values that, for generations, had served as a compass for guiding human action. Gone were the old bench marks that had given us our sense of identity and that we had come to rely upon in times of uncertainty and trouble—the teachings of the church, loyalty and dedication to one's family, a sense of purpose and meaning in one's work. With the old value system eroded and with nothing to take its place, we entered a period of nervousness and uncertainty characterized as the twentieth-century "age of anxiety." Interestingly enough, physicians were among the first to observe this important change. Why so? Because their consulting rooms began to fill with patients whose physical problems were now compounded by a new set of difficulties—feelings of chronic anxiety, tension, and fatigue. And even the best physicians were hard pressed to find physical explanations for much of this malaise and discontent. As we moved through the halfway mark of the century into the mid 1970s, family physicians were reporting, almost with unanimity, that in addition to whatever medical problems their patients might bring, well over 50 per cent were suffering from varying degrees of emotional depletion—boredom, loneliness, and absence of purpose and direction in their lives. Chronic fatigue was the common manifestation of this new problem.

It is in this setting then that this guideline on dealing with fatigue appears. And I am happy to report that it is a most useful guide indeed. Linda Pembrook is a perceptive and skilled writer and she has done her homework well. She has thoroughly researched a fascinating, though complicated, medical subject and she presents an authoritative up-to-date review of what we know about the causes and cures of fatigue. She has gone to the experts and literally picked their brains for the best advice currently available. As a result, these pages are filled with sound practical recommendations that will help the reader spot possible physical causes of fatigue and will alert him to signs and symptoms of illnesses that may require the attention of a physician. It also provides a clear and understandable description of the many psychological states that commonly result in tension, anxiousness, and chronic tiredness. Most important this is a book on how to conquer fatigue and, for this reason, it should be helpful to doctors (themselves no strangers to fatigue) and patients alike. It outlines step-by-step approaches for coming to grips with the most common emotional traps that result in fatigue, and the advice given is both practical and sound. Above all it works! Read this book carefully, follow its program of instruction, and you will gain immense benefit in renewed energy and enjoyment of life.

Donald T. Fredrickson, M.D.
Inter-Society Commission for Heart
Diseases Resources
January 1975

How to beat fatigue

PART ONE

Physical fatigue

Like those enviable folks who apparently can eat to their hearts' desire without gaining an ounce, there is also the person who seems endlessly to recharge himself with energy, who is always on the go and never late getting there.

Many public figures seem blessed with this endless vitality. How, one wonders, can a particular politician spend the afternoon addressing a women's organization in Cleveland, the evening attending a fund-raising dinner in Chicago, and the following morning receiving an honorary degree in Seattle? And to what degree does his professional success reflect his ability to withstand fatigue?

Energy is the vital ingredient without which we do not feel quite fully alive. No matter how many pleasures surround us, we need energy in order to enjoy them. To the person who is tired, a lively book may be boring, a delicious meal mediocre, a beautiful day uninteresting. Moreover, the person whose energy level is low and whose spirits are faded is not very much fun to be with.

Most people don't need to be told that life would take on brighter colors if they could inject more vitality into it. But is such a transformation conceivable? Is one born with a certain energy level to which one must adapt? Or is it possible to breathe new life into collapsing sails?

The answer, fortunately, is the latter: It is possible to replenish your personal fuel reserves, to work a harder day and yet enjoy leisure time more.

This book is aimed primarily at people who are chronically tired and who perhaps have been searching for years for the reason. In the process they may have swallowed tons of vitamin pills or drunk gallons of whiskey in an effort to "pick themselves up." They have read hundreds of articles on fatigue, and some have dragged themselves from one doctor to another in search of a solution.

The book is also for people for whom fatigue is not an overwhelming problem which cuts heavily into their enjoyment of life, but merely a recurring and annoying phenomenon which keeps them from feeling in top condition as often as they would like.

Both chronic and temporary fatigue frequently have a psychological component—boredom, anxiety, stress, depression. But not necessarily so. It is possible to be fatigued simply because you drink too much, you don't get enough exercise, you don't sleep well, you have an undiagnosed illness, you aren't eating the proper foods, or you don't make good use of your time.

This book will discuss both the physiological and the psychological components of fatigue. The distinction is somewhat arbitrary, because in many cases the two are difficult to separate. For example, a person who is in a constant state of anxiety may not be eating a nourishing diet, and the two factors play against each other to augment the fatigue. Likewise, someone who is sleeping poorly may find himself more susceptible to stress.

Usually, however, either a psychological or a physiological cause will predominate, whether a person is tired all the time or merely too often for comfort. In either case, the cure lies in finding the cause. Very possibly, you can make the diagnosis yourself, then decide whether or not you need the help of a doctor. If poor circulation from lack of exercise is chiefly at fault, you can easily set up your own exercise regime. If your fatigue is the consequence of an overburdened emotional life, professional counseling may be the answer.

Before concentrating on the major causes of fatigue, let's take a look at some obvious possibilities. Is your tiredness possibly due to the fact that your shoes don't fit properly, or your office chair is the wrong height?

Various physiological conditions can produce fatigue—for instance, lack of oxygen. Anyone who has taken a mountain vacation has noted that he is ready for bed earlier at a high elevation. A lack of salt, water, or sugar also create physiological imbalances that result in fatigue. The reason we feel tired after a long period of not eating is that our blood sugar level has dropped.

High temperatures cause fatigue, as someone who has been sitting for a long time in an overheated room can testify. People who work in poorly ventilated places also tire more quickly.

Once these fairly obvious causes of fatigue have been eliminated, you can begin to probe more deeply. A note of warning: Answers will not necessarily come at once, since fatigue may result from a complex combination of factors, some of them obscure. Prepare, therefore, to step back and take the long view, regarding fatigue not as an isolated phenomenon, but within the context of your internal and external life.

I DEFINING FATIGUE

"Fatigue, like anxiety, relatively permanent impairment, and illness or disease, is a form of human inadequacy," notes Dr. S. Howard Bartley, one of the country's foremost authorities on the subject. "All of these everyday terms lack precision and distinction, and definition is, therefore, a fundamental problem."

For many years it was thought that fatigue was a condition exclusive to people who had been working too hard. Investigators began to analyze the efforts of factory workers and to try to correlate them with degrees of tiredness. These early industrial psychologists and engineers were puzzled, however, by their inability to draw parallels between the amount of work someone accomplished and how he said he felt. Some workers put out prodigious amounts and reported themselves feeling fine; others were "exhausted" after unexceptional efforts.

Further research revealed that muscular activity causes the consumption of oxygen and glucose (blood sugar) and the excretion of carbon dioxide and uric acid. This line of analysis was used particularly in studies of athletes or heavy laborers, where attempts were made to quantify energy. Till recently, little thought was given to the fact that many demands other than physical ones can produce fatigue. Not all activity is muscular; the brain, too, gets tired.

Dr. Bartley offers the following observations about fatigue:

• Fatigue comes and goes throughout the day, and we do not always feel as tired at night as in the morning;

• We can wake up in the morning after a full night's sleep and feel more tired than when we went to bed;

• We become more tired doing something unpleasant than something enjoyable;

• Though worn out from a day at work, we can dance energetically all night or play nine holes of golf the same evening;

• If a particular chore is tiring the first time we attempt it, it will be tiring the next time too;

• People cannot always pinpoint exactly what it is that makes them tired.

These observations affirm that theories which link fatigue solely with energy loss are not very useful, Dr. Bartley points out. "If fatigue is depletion of energy, it is something that happens to the cells of the body, primarily the muscle cells. If depletion of energy resources in these cells occurs, one could not expect energy to be restored until more food is eaten or else some stored supply is released."

Dr. Bartley's conclusion is that the term *fatigue* describes a personal experience—a sort of self-evaluation—rather than a state of muscle tissue. For example, recently the owner of a men's clothing store woke up and immediately started thinking about everything that had to be done at the shop. Inventory was still not completed, two clerks were quitting, and vandals had cracked one of his store windows. Also, he worried that an expensive new line of shirts might not sell. Suddenly he felt tired, and the sensations in his muscles testified to this feeling.

But suddenly he was struck by a dazzling realization—it was Sunday morning, not Saturday, and the shop was closed. He was free to roll over and go back to sleep. Immediately those bodily sensations took on a different meaning. Instead of representing unpleasant tiredness, they represented relaxation and the absence of tension.

Frequently one feels much more tired after a night of deep sleep than after a night of tossing and turning. Dr. Bartley suggests that just as we must leave our tensions behind in order to go to sleep, we need to regain a certain amount of muscular tension in order to get out of bed feeling alert. "Deep sleep could well result in a lower level of muscle tone than a lighter sleep and would therefore require a greater amount of time to build up tone to a fully adequate level," he explains.

In summary, fatigue is not an objective measure of individual energy resources. "The human organism is continually expressing an orientation to the environment," Dr. Bartley comments. "As I see it, fatigue is the name for the highest level of this expression, namely, the conscious individual's self-assessment of his feelings of aversion to and inadequacy for carrying on in a responsible way."

Mental attitude is crucial

According to studies currently in progress at the University of Wisconsin, different individuals use up various amounts of energy doing the same thing, depending on how they regard the task. If Harry believes that push-ups are exhausting, he may exert the same amount of energy to perform ten push-ups that Ernest, a sports enthusiast, uses to push himself up and down fifteen times.

Dr. William Morgan, who heads the research unit, feels that much of our daily fatigue is a product of poor assessment of our capabilities, and that it may be possible to increase productivity by simply re-evaluating the task at hand.

"If we can learn more about work-rest cycles," he points out, "possibly people will be able to work at more optimum perceived exertion levels."

He is particularly interested in the possibility of applying results to the treatment of cardiac patients, many of whom hesitate to carry out their prescribed exercises for fear of becoming exhausted. If the perceptions of these patients could be changed, their tolerance would increase, says Dr. Morgan.

The phenomenon of "second wind" is also one which has interested people for a long time. For example, a college student sits down unenthusiastically to a night of writing a term paper. Although at first his attitude is stale, gradually he warms up to the job and eventually even becomes interested.

After four hours he feels the level of his fatigue rising, and he is ready to quit. However, a third of the paper remains unwritten. Plugging along, he suddenly finds that his fatigue has evaporated, and that he in fact has found a second wind, which propels him the rest of the way through the paper. Somehow he has tapped a new layer of energy.

According to William James, the famous psychologist and philosopher of the nineteenth century, most of us could easily push through this fatigue barrier more often. "Everyone knows that on any given day there are energies slumbering in him which the incitements of that day do not call forth," he comments. "Compared with what we ought to be, we are only half awake. Our fires are damped, our drafts are checked. We are making use of only a small part of our possible mental and physical resources."

Only exceptional individuals are willing to push to their extremes, he points out, while most of us are content to remain a step behind our potential capabilities. These exceptional people can be spurred either by emotional excitement which urges them onwards or by some necessity that demands an extra effort of will.

The kind of person who is able to push through a physiologic energy barrier is often the one who is capable of great personal growth, says James.

Frequently, when one accepts a position of greater responsibility, he surprises both himself and others by his new-found zest for working and changing.

The call of duty can also bring to fruition the talents and capabilities of ordinary citizens. For instance, a woman who is suddenly widowed will often show much more moral fiber than people ever gave her credit for. Suddenly she is forced to take on all the responsibility and direction of the household, in addition to everything she was doing before. Her new life may leave her exhausted physically and mentally, but somewhere she must find the strength to continue.

"Despair, which lames most people, wakes others fully up," James observes. "Every siege or shipwreck or polar expedition brings out some hero who keeps the whole company in heart."

He offers the example of an explosion in a French coal mine many years ago which left two hundred people dead. After twenty days of excavation, when the victims' families were abandoning hope, the rescuers heard a faint voice. The man calling out had taken charge of thirteen others in the darkness, disciplined and cheered them, and brought them out alive.

Of course, most people do not have the misfortune of being buried in a coal mine, or something similarly dramatic, to force their bodies beyond the normal physiological shutoff point. The customary way of digging deeper and deeper into energy reserves is by effort of will.

"A single successful effort of moral volition, such as saying no to some habitual temptation, or performing some courageous act, will launch a man on a higher level of energy for days and weeks, will give him a new range of power," James promises.

Dieters could certainly confirm this theory: The first time a tempting dessert is pushed away, the dieter senses a rising exaltation which often carries him through to the next courageous act of refusal. Likewise the heavy drinker: The first time he shuns the proffered bottle, life can take on whole new dimensions.

James feels that healthy people can push their energies to an extreme every day and suffer no ill effects. "A man's more active rate of energizing does not wreck him, for the organism adapts itself," he says. "As the rate of waste augments, so does the rate of repair."

People who habitually put in long hours of work usually need no more sleep than those who sit around doing next to nothing. And a busy man will find that he probably sleeps the same amount of time while on vacation in the mountains as when back in the city. In fact, he may sleep longer on vacation, when there is no urgent reason to get up.

Thus, according to James, "the human individual usually lives far within his limits. In rough terms," he adds critically, "we may say that a man who energizes below his normal maximum fails by just so much to profit by his chance at life."

Studies of airline pilots

William James had a lot of wise thoughts, but he died in 1910 and thus never had to come to grips with the frustrations of life in the 1970s.

Many studies of the physiology of fatigue have been made under the auspices of large industries, which are looking for ways to increase the production of their workers. Usually these studies are based on "artificial" fatigue induced in the laboratory and not observed as a natural occurrence.

One exception was an examination carried out in Australia a few years ago at the instigation of the workers themselves—in this case, airline pilots who were suffering prolonged fatigue. Author of the study, Dr. C. Cameron of the Australian Road Research Board, concluded that simple physical fatigue is a disminishing problem in this world, while the more complex phenomenon of mental fatigue is on the rise.

Results of the airline study are particularly valid, he stresses, because the artificiality of the standard fatigue analyses has been screened out. "It is well known that attempts to measure fatigue objectively are often frustrated by what are usually called 'motivational factors,'" he explains. "The subject in fatigue experiments seems to be able to resist performance decrement by making an extra effort. The difficulty here is to determine the relevance of such results to actual work performance."

The investigation took place in two phases: first, a sample group of sixty pilots was thoroughly examined, through a lengthy technical interview, and later by a specialist in aviation medicine. Pilots' wives were also interviewed. Researchers then accompanied the pilots on observation flights. Later, questionnaires were sent to six hundred pilots to confirm and help evaluate the material collected from the original group.

Although other efforts had concentrated mainly on the performance aspects of behavior, this one explored the subjective state of the individual.

Dr. Cameron concluded from the study that fatigue is a state not of low arousal, but of high arousal. The tired airline pilots showed much evidence of chronic over-arousal; 25 per cent complained of frequent indigestion or stomach upset, another 25 per cent suffered milder gastric symptoms. Prolonged fatigue produced sleep disturbance as well as other symptoms of stress such as increased drinking and smoking, irritability, and general restlessness.

Clinically speaking, they resembled people suffering a mild anxiety state. "It would be overstating the case to describe them as sufferers from anxiety neurosis," Dr. Cameron observes, "but it would be accurate to describe them as people who spend a large proportion of time feeling something less than 100 per cent fit, and who have to make a constant effort to cope with the demands of their daily lives."

Deterioration in the performance of pilots was demonstrated some years ago in the Cambridge, England, "Cockpit Studies." A large group of RAF pilots were required to "fly" for at least two hours under simulated conditions, some continuing for six to seven hours till they were exhausted.

Although errors due to the misuse of controls declined steadily throughout the experiments, this improvement was more than counterbalanced by a loss of accuracy of timing and skill. As subjects became increasingly tired, they were willing to settle for lower and lower standards of accuracy and performance.

In addition, they were unable to interpret the various instrument readings as part of a single integrated system, but focused on one reading as an individual, isolated instrument. As time went on, they might forget about some of the instruments not directly in front of them.

Most interesting: As they approached the end of a flight, they made more and more mistakes. Apparently, a tired pilot has an almost irresistible tendency to take it easy when the airport is in sight.

"In skill fatigue, then, the 'standards' accepted and followed by the central nervous system unwittingly deteriorate," Dr. McFarland points out. "Although a person may think he is doing better work, actually his performance is getting poorer and poorer. At first, it is more likely that he will do the right things at the wrong time, but if accurate timing is important, gross errors will finally begin to appear."

On-the-job-fatigue

Airline pilots represent a small slice of the world's population, but the Australian study pointed up a few things worth noting in our technological society. For one thing, it revealed the existence of chronic sleep disturbances in people working on night shifts.

As an industry becomes more automated, Dr. Cameron points

out, it becomes less tolerant of variation in the personal preferences and established work habits of its employees. Although a humane man-machine system could be designed, he feels, no one has attempted one. What often results, then, is "a system which makes excessive demands on the physical and mental capabilities of the men and women who have to work in it. The workers have to make the effort of adaptation."

It has been shown more than once that when the working day is lengthened, hourly productivity goes down; conversely, when people are allowed to work a shorter day, they put more into each hour.

For example, during the Battle of Britain in World War II, when the British were under the continuing menace of German attack, factories went on a 24-hour-a-day, 7-day-a-week schedule. At first, patriotism produced a surge in production. After a few months, however, factory managers began to notice an increase in illness, absenteeism, and tardiness. Yet when Sunday was rescheduled as a day of rest, production did not fall off. In fact, one factory set a new weekly record.

Economic analysts concluded that beyond a certain maximum point, which varies with each industry, increased hours of work do not equal more production and may even mean less.

Dr. McFarland suggests that for most industries in the United States, the standard eight-hour working day represents the limit of productivity. "For easier work or where it is possible to schedule several relaxing breaks over the course of the work day, longer hours may well be permissible," he adds.

People working day shifts consistently produce more and with many less errors than those on the night shift, studies have shown. The explanation seems to be that the night shift is incompatible with our circadian rhythm. Nighttime workers feel disoriented and out of tune with both the hour and with each other.

In summary, then, it is not possible to draw parallels between fatigue and energy expenditure. Muscular exertion produces biochemical changes in the body that can give rise to stiffness and tiredness, and a person who has overexerted himself will usually feel the effects. On the other hand, it is possible to be physiologically fatigued—for instance, after conducting an orchestra for several hours—yet feel exhilarated rather than tired.

This is because fatigue is also an expression of a person's assessment of a situation. If he doesn't like what he is doing, is uncomfortable doing it, or fears failure, his brain will communicate the fact to his body. Physical and emotional processes are integrally related, although the interaction is not clearly understood.

BIBLIOGRAPHY

Bartley, S. Howard. "Fatigue," *Encyclopaedia Britannica,* 1974.

————. "What Do You Mean, 'Tired'?" *Today's Education,* Feb. 1969.

Cameron, C. "Fatigue Problems in Modern Industry," *Ergonomics,* 1971, vol. 14, no. 6.

"It's How It Seems That Counts," *Medical World News,* Apr. 6, 1973.

James, William. "How to Increase Your Energy," *Reader's Digest,* Sept. 1971.

McFarland, R. A. "Understanding Fatigue in Modern Life," *Ergonomics,* 1971, vol. 14, no. 1.

2 GETTING CONTROL OF TIME

Our sense of well-being is influenced not only by mental and physical health, but by the time of day. In fact, many misunderstandings occur and false accusations are hurled as a result of people's failure to appreciate the wide variations in individual body rhythms.

For example, George discovers that his new wife Gerry has absolutely no intention of fixing breakfast for the two of them in the morning. She dozes away till he has finished shaving, staggers out of bed, and throws herself together to go to work.

George, on the other hand, is always the first to start yawning at a dinner party. Almost the minute the last bite of dessert has been swallowed and coffee cups are being refilled, his eyes start traveling to the door.

George is not antisocial, nor is his wife lazy. Their circadian rhythms—the built-in timing device that is attuned to the 24-hour turn of the earth—are very different. George feels great first thing in the morning; Gerry comes alive at cocktail hour.

Understanding your own body clock can be a very effective way of fighting fatigue. If you understand your cycle, you will plan to be most active during the high periods, and try to avoid knocking yourself out at the low points. The following questions should be of help:

· How do you feel when you wake up? Is your day a gradual process of awakening, or do you jump eagerly from bed and wind down from there on?

· On vacations or weekends, what time do you go to bed and what time do you get up?

· What time of day are you happiest, and when are you likely to feel low?

· When do you like to make love?

· Do drugs affect you differently at different times of the day?

· When do you eat your biggest meal?

In the urban environment to which most of us are accustomed, the forces of nature seem almost irrelevant. We control our own world, independent of everything except our own body functions.

Yet even in the twentieth century, we have not lost touch with the cosmos. As Gay Gaer Luce writes about New Yorkers, living in a round-the-clock city where bars are still doing business and buses running at 4 A.M., "While we sometimes act as if we are capable of machine-like flexibility, we cannot act that way very often or very long except at our peril. We are giant, living clocks, part of the larger clock of the rotating earth we live upon, which is, in turn, part of the rhythmic change of our solar system, of our galaxy."

Probably, she points out, one of the main ways that primitive organisms survived on this earth was by adapting to rhythm. Because sunlight could be converted into plant energy, these organisms may have attuned themselves to the 24-hour, day-and-night rotation of the earth. We human beings have inherited that circadian rhythm, no matter where we live.

Most obviously, the circadian rhythm influences us when we go to sleep. It also influences body temperature (which goes up during the day and drops a degree or two at night) and body functions. Blood pressure, mood, pulse, respiration, blood sugar levels, amino acid levels, and the ability to metabolize drugs, all follow a rising and falling pattern.

"Levels of crucial hormones in our blood and concentrations of essential brain chemicals mean that there is a subtle rhythm to the efficiency with which we metabolize food, to the quickness of our reaction time, to the keenness of our sensory perception and discrimination," Ms. Luce points out.

Round-the-clock cities won't work

Numbers of employees choose, or are obliged to work, hours deemed unacceptable to most of the population: the policeman who works a midnight to 9 A.M. shift, the night watchman, the bus driver who sees the sun rise every morning and is in bed before it sets.

As long as such schedules are regular, health does not seem to be affected. It is the irregular shifts that give rise to ulcers and other symptoms of stress. For example, pilots and stewardesses on an east-west run have great difficulty adjusting their internal time clocks to earth time, and evidence suggests that they age faster than the rest of us.

If a city were converted officially to a 24-hour schedule, with stores and schools open, offices functioning, restaurants serving at all hours, the incidence of neurosis would shoot up immediately. We all need a time of quiet, for sleeping, dreaming, and psychically renewing ourselves without the interruptions of a daytime existence.

As Ms. Luce points out, "No man is a closed system, and no technology can protect us from other invisible rhythms of our earth and space around it. These are gravitational changes, changes in electromagnetic fields, barometric pressure changes, cascades of cosmic rays."

It has been observed many times that when the moon is full, crimes of violence rise, and the inmates of psychiatric hospitals begin to stir. No one can fully explain this phenomenon, or other ones concerning man's relationship with his universe. Clearly, however, there are influences working upon us of which we are only vaguely aware.

Light, for example, does more than allow us to see; it acts as a synchronizer of the circadian rhythm and apparently activates the adrenal glands. Birds use light to tell them when to migrate and when to mate; they are somehow attuned to the changing ratio between light and darkness in the progression of seasons.

Experiments where people have dwelt in caves voluntarily for long periods have demonstrated the importance of light in synchronizing activity and internal rhythm with day and night. These cave dwellers find that their normal rhythm is broken after even short spells in darkness, and that they are not living a 24-hour cycle.

Light also has an effect on the menstrual cycle; biologists have been able to prevent ovulation in female rats merely by giving them light at a critical time of the month. The human menstrual cycle has also shown itself responsive to light.

Gaining control of your time

The majority of Americans slog through life without even considering how they are spending their time. Everything is taken for granted: work time, leisure time, travel time, sleep time.

When we do something outside its normal time slot, we often feel guilty or uneasy. To take an extra hour at lunch in order to enjoy a beautiful day is like stealing from the company, even if the consequent rise in spirits makes for a more productive afternoon. Many people go to bed at the same hour all their lives, tired or not, out of sheer force of habit.

The relationship between how a person spends his time and his energy levels is a crucial one. According to Alan Lakein, a time management consultant who has studied his subject extensively, there is always time to do what is important and still have plenty of room for relaxation.

"Can you work effectively if you are too fatigued from excessive hours?" he asks. "Probably not. Maybe a better solution would be to quit early, take the afternoon and evening off, and come back the next day refreshed and physically able to work twice as hard."

Large corporations have been using management consultants for years to find more productive ways of using their employees, improving morale, and increasing production. Now those techniques are being made available to the private individual.

Mr. Lakein first asks a new client to consider: When you say you want to use your time more productively, what kind of time do you mean? A minute from now, or the next hour, the next month, or your whole life?

"Most people operate in the mid-range of mediocrity, in the range of hours or days," he maintains. "They don't think in terms of minutes—the little chunks most time comes in. They waste all the minutes."

Nor do these people look ahead to a whole year or a whole lifetime, he adds. "Essentially they start over every week, and spend another chunk unrelated to their lifetime goals. They are doing a random walk through life, moving without getting anywhere."

People "on the way up" are particularly likely to allow their family and personal lives to be drained by work demands. Often they are so goal-oriented that they feel guilty about taking time for anything not in some way related to earning a living.

Mr. Lakein tells the story of an architect who, only days after recovering from a bleeding ulcer, was back at the drafting board sixty hours a week, and complaining that he didn't see enough of his wife and children.

After much urging, the architect was persuaded to leave work regularly at 5 P.M. and also at noon on Fridays. Then he would head with his family for a cabin on a lake, without briefcase. Forced to concentrate only on essential matters at work, he managed to pack a tremendous amount into the hours that he did spend there, relegating some of the detail he had previously engulfed himself in to the staff. Not surprisingly, he found that some of his most creative thoughts occurred during quiet moments with a fishing rod.

Many people have to be taught how to "relax and do nothing"; their leisure hours are as filled with activity and as tightly scheduled as their working days. Paula, a young interior decorator from Connecticut, complained recently that the ski weekends she and her boyfriend spent in Vermont last winter were more of an endurance test than a pleasure. After a four-hour drive on a Friday night, they would go out to dinner with the other two couples sharing the house, then crash exhausted into bed around midnight.

Next morning everybody was up at the crack of dawn cooking breakfast and preparing for a long day on the slopes. "The lift tickets are expensive, so John felt he had to ski every minute to get his money's worth," his girl friend explains. "If the skiing wasn't good, we'd spend the entire day driving all over the state bargain-hunting for antiques."

Sunday night the couple arrived back home weary, wet, and exhausted after a long drive. Getting up on Monday morning, bones aching, was an agony.

"One season was enough, even for John," Paula relates. "I convinced him that we'd be better off taking three solid weeks of skiing in one place—maybe Switzerland—and spending our winter weekends reading books and going to the movies. Frankly, I love to just sit by a fire, relax, and do nothing."

Listing your priorities

Mr. Lakein feels that pencil and paper are essential to any long-range planning and reorganization of life; when people are forced to put their thoughts into words, they get a better idea of what they really want.

First question: What are your lifetime goals? Fill up an entire sheet of paper as quickly as possible with every conceivable thing you would like to do—money, career, physical, family, social, community, spiritual, and personal goals. Make no effort to assign priorities: "lose five pounds, visit Russia, fix the bird feeder, develop rapport with my sister, and get a new job" should all go, at random, on the same list.

When you have finished, place an *A* in front of three goals that seem most important. With a new sheet of paper, allow two minutes per item for writing down as many subgoals as possible: How will goal *A* be accomplished? What is the first step?

Next, select one item from each *A* goal and force yourself to start the wheels in motion the following week. Each month, take out pencil and paper and make a new list. Only by having a few clearly identified goals in life can you hope to make headway in achieving them.

The second question in the pencil-paper game: How would you like to spend the next five years? In answering this, think about the things you really want to do, not what you have been told to want.

If you answer, "I want to make a lot of money and become secure in my profession" or "I want to get married," you may be speaking for your parents, but not for yourself. A more honest answer might be, "I'd like to move to someplace where the weather is warmer" or "I'd like to get a divorce" or "I want to finish law school."

It is easy to let the next five years roll along in their predictable fashion, but it is also possible to give some shape to your life despite obligations and limitations. If you can recognize certain things that you want, you will be much more likely to take them into consideration when making major decisions.

The complaint is frequently heard that "I'd like to, but it's out of the question . . . I'm too old" or "I don't have the money" or "I don't have the time." Unfortunately, many timid souls are bound much more by their own lack of imagination than by limitations imposed from outside. The mere act of making a list pulls at least slightly on imaginative reserves, and it presents a tangible object to confront which contains at least a few real possibilities. Hang it on your closet door or keep it in your top desk drawer.

Third and last question: How would you like to live if you knew you would be dead in six months? Some people are so out of touch with themselves that they have never seriously considered what it is they enjoy in life. Again, once they have organized their thoughts and put them down on paper, choices can be made.

How an expert does it

Mr. Lakein, whose past clients include IBM, Standard Oil of California, and AT&T, and who has incorporated his expertise into a book, keeps a check on his own time as follows:

1. I don't own a television set. My family and I went to a motel to watch the moonwalks and we rented a set for the political conventions.

2. I skim books quickly, looking for ideas.

3. I have my office close enough to my home to be able to walk to work.

4. I've given up forever all "waiting time." If I have to wait I consider it a "gift of time" to relax, plan or do something I would not otherwise have done.

5. I keep my watch three minutes fast.

6. I revise my life-goals list once a month.

7. I carry blank three-by-five index cards in my pocket to jot down notes and ideas.

8. I put up signs reminding me of my goals.

9. I schedule my time months in advance in such a way that each month offers variety and balance as well as "open time" reserved for "hot" projects.

10. I give myself time off and special rewards when I've done the important things.

11. If I seem to procrastinate, I ask myself: "What am I avoiding?" And then I try to confront that thing head-on.

12. I start with the most profitable parts of large projects, and often find it is not necessary to do the rest.

13. I do much of my thinking on paper.

14. I work alone creatively in the mornings and use the afternoons for meetings.

15. I save all trivia for a three-hour session once a month.

16. I delegate everything I possibly can.

17. I make use of specialists to help me with special problems.

18. I keep a list of specific items to be done each day, arrange them in priority order, and then do my best to get the important ones done as soon as possible.

19. I generate as little paper work as possible and throw away anything I possibly can.

20. I handle each piece of paper only once.

21. I write replies to most letters right on the piece of paper.

22. I set deadlines for myself and others.

23. I try not to think of work on weekends.

24. I "do nothing" rather frequently.

How to fight jet lag

In this age of jet travel, many people know what it is like to feel out of sorts for days after traveling through several time zones. How distressing to nod through dinner in a London restaurant, then to wake up at 4 A.M. ready to go sightseeing.

By shifting the hours of sleep, we desynchronize a vast number of internal cycles, and maladjusted sleep is the most visible proof. Some organs seem to adjust faster than others; thus a person may be working with a body that is still asleep and whose hormone levels are low, or sleeping with a body that is still ready to function at maximum capacity.

Jet lag affects people in varying degrees. Some people are able to adjust with only a minimum of discomfort. The popular rule of thumb is that it takes one day of adjustment for each hour of difference in time. Many people can bounce to their feet more quickly than that.

Here are a few suggestions to help jump the hurdle:

• Eat moderately before, during, and after the flight. If you eat everything the airline serves you, and in addition keep to the meal schedule back home and in the place you are headed, you will be very uncomfortable.

• Don't take a sleeping pill, the effects of which will not wear off before you deplane. Instead, count sheep, or listen to the drone of the engine.

• Try to keep as closely as possible to the hours in the new place. Force yourself to stay awake till evening so that you fall asleep tired. If sleep is elusive, now is the time for a sleeping pill to help get your cycle into gear.

For people who work too hard

Undeniably, there are people in this world for whom fatigue is a simple consequence of overwork. A young mother has four pre-school children, a house to clean, meals to prepare. More nights than not, she drops into a chair exhausted when the last dish has been wiped—only then she has some mending to do before morning. An artist takes on several projects at once and finds they demand much more time than he had estimated. His wife is ill, and on top of everything else he has to shoulder household and child-rearing duties.

Most people know when they are working too hard, because their thoughts are constantly preoccupied with the tasks at hand and the limited time available for accomplishing them. Other people, however, may not realize that they have bitten off more than they can chew. A man in his sixties may not recognize that he cannot maintain the pace he set as a young man. He jogs for an hour in the morning, puts in a full day at the office, comes home for a few rounds of cocktails, then sets off for a lengthy formal dinner. No wonder he's often tired.

Unfortunately, there are no easy cures for the exhaustion that results from necessary constant overexertion—except, where feasible, to take it easy. It is possible, however, to take some of the stresses out of the working situation.

Factory owners have found that workers tire less easily and are more productive when they are supplied with background music and when they are allowed frequent short breaks. The housewife might also think in those terms. Instead of leaving the TV blaring after the children have seen the last of the morning cartoons, she might put on the waltzes of Chopin or the soft sounds of a Spanish guitar. Rather than wait till 9 P.M. to collapse, she might take a half-hour nap after lunch.

Harassed people could control their time better if they only understood how different types of work take different tolls of energy. Obviously, difficult, frustrating, or repetitive jobs are more tiring than other kinds, and jobs that one hates to do should be scheduled for those times when morale and energy levels are high.

The business person who finds correspondence a chore should tap out a few letters first thing in the morning. The college student who loathes biology should open the biology book right after lunch, if that is when he feels best. The point is: Analyze what it is that your job requires of you, and try to arrange it in the least tiring fashion.

BIBLIOGRAPHY

Lakein, Alan. *How to Get Control of Your Time and Your Life,* Peter H. Wyden, 1973.

Luce, Gay Gaer. "Understanding Body Time in the 24-Hour City," *New York Magazine,* Nov. 15, 1971.

O'Reilly, Jane. "How to Get Control of Your Time (and Your Life)," *New York Magazine,* Jan. 17, 1972.

Wyatt, Richard. "Are You Getting Enough Sleep?" *U.S. News & World Report,* Oct. 16, 1972.

3 HOW MUCH SLEEP IS ENOUGH?

"You look tired—you need a good eight hours sleep." This is a time-worn and apparently logical piece of advice that is becoming more and more suspect. Recent research suggests, first, that fatigue is frequently no barometer of lack of sleep, and second, that eight hours is no magic number in any case.

For some time now, researchers have been shooting holes in many of the familiar theories about sleep—exactly what happens in the process, who needs how much, and how people react when deprived of sleep.

Most of us spend a third of our lives sleeping. Scientifically, the term *sleep* denotes a state of inactivity and muscular relaxation, when normal sensory stimuli such as the touch of a hand or the sound of a passing car produce no conscious reaction. Poets and novelists have made much of the healing powers of sleep, although even today we are not sure how it "knits up the ravel'd sleave of care."

Despite age-old curiosity about sleep and dreams, no one investigated sleep under laboratory conditions until the late 1930s. No one had actually watched a person go to sleep and recorded his observations scientifically. Some studies were published in the early part of this century, but they were based on what volunteer subjects themselves said about their sleeping and dreaming experiences, not on what the researchers observed.

It was about thirty-five years ago that Dr. Nathaniel Kleitman of the University of Chicago set up the first sleep laboratory and launched the research which has since been pursued by others. One of his earliest discoveries was that, despite the claims of people who always "sleep like a log," most of us shift positions many times during the night.

In 1952 Dr. Kleitman and his coworkers evolved the laboratory techniques which laid the groundwork for the many sleep studies being carried out today. One of the earliest myths shattered was the belief that all dreams last only a few seconds. The investigators found that when a person dreams he is flying for five minutes, for example, the dream actually lasts for five minutes. Real time and perceived time are the same.

Before sleep research, it was thought that endomorphs—soft, plump people—like to sleep and therefore go to sleep more easily and sleep more deeply, while thin, high-strung people—ectomorphs —have trouble sleeping because they would rather be out doing something active. The basic premise of this theory—that there may be built-in, genetically determined predispositions to sleep well or poorly—has not been totally discounted, but the issue is not as cut-and-dried as investigators had hoped.

Psychological study
New insights into the question of what kind of people sleep longest and why are supplied by a recent co-operative study conducted at Tufts University School of Medicine in Boston and Downstate Medical Center in Brooklyn. In an analysis of more than three hundred male volunteers over age twenty, the researchers came to the conclusion that men who consistently sleep less than six hours per night are generally efficient people who tend to handle stress by denying

it and keeping busy. Long sleepers (more than nine hours) are worrying types, chronically somewhat depressed or anxious.

"Almost all long sleepers had a positive attitude towards sleep, that is, they valued it highly and thought it was important," notes psychiatrist Dr. Ernest Hartmann, director of the study and a well-known sleep authority. "Short sleepers either had a negative attitude towards sleep or felt neutral."

Dr. Hartmann also found that short sleepers tolerated sleep loss considerably better than their opposites. In general, they were more extroverted, had higher energy levels, and were more ambitious. Long sleepers were more likely to have a lower than normal sex drive.

During the testing, long sleepers fretted much more about laboratory conditions, complaining about temperature in the room, the quality of the beds, and irritation from the electrodes placed on their heads. Short sleepers seemed relatively sure of themselves, socially adept, decisive, satisfied with themselves and their lives.

"They had few complaints either about the study, about their life situation, or about politics and the state of the world," Dr. Hartmann reports. "They were somewhat conformist in their social and political views, and they wished to appear very normal and 'all American.' They seldom left themselves time to sit down and think about problems; in fact, several of them, on being asked what they did in times of stress or worry, made statements such as, 'I never let my worries go to my head.'"

Few of these volunteers had any problems which would land them on a psychiatrist's couch. If there was anything "wrong" with them, it was that they bent over backwards to avoid problems. Long sleepers were a little harder to pigeonhole. They revealed a wide range of opinions on all subjects, tending to be nonconformist and critical in their social and political views. Most had moderate neurotic disturbances.

Generally, these people appeared not very sure of themselves, their career choices, or their life styles, although several were fairly well-established in creative fields. A few admitted that they sometimes used sleep as an escape when reality was unpleasant. Overall, the long sleepers were definitely worriers who quickly let problems assume vast dimensions, Dr. Hartmann stresses.

Although the differences between long and short sleepers were marked, Dr. Hartmann cautions that no hard lines can be drawn between sleep need and personality make-up. "Possibly, certain personalities and life styles produce a requirement for more sleep than others. On the other hand, sleeping long hours may bring on certain character changes, and sleeping short hours other ones. A third possibility: Certain genetic patterns may produce quite independently both a low requirement for sleep and a hypomanic life style. I tend to back the first alternative."

Discovering the fundamentals

The big breakthrough in sleep studies came in 1952, when Dr. Kleitman's experiments with an electroencephalograph (EEG) machine disclosed the existence of four stages of sleep. These stages were found to progress evenly in rhythmical cycles that continue through the night, and one stage is characterized by dreaming.

Traditionally, sleep was considered a time of total unconsciousness and inactivity, when worn body tissues were repaired and worn-out cells replaced. Now we know that body tissues restore themselves while we are awake; in fact, healthy people function best when their daytime life is active and their intervals of rest brief. Researchers suggest that even when a person is asleep, periodic muscle movements prevent total muscular inactivity.

While sleep had always been regarded as a time when the weary brain ground to a halt, EEG measurements show that the brain is in fact far from inert at night; rather, it consistently emits electrical impulses which change according to how deeply the person is sleeping. Although the brain's activity changes in form at night, the amount of activity does not decrease.

Researchers have divided sleep into four phases according to the changes in brain waves. When a person is awake, his EEG is characterized by the so-called alpha rhythm brain waves, which have a frequency of about ten cycles per second. As the subject falls asleep, the alpha rhythm often disappears and reappears a few times, then is gradually lost.

For the first ten minutes or so after he falls asleep, he continues to be aware of his surroundings and would claim to be still awake if asked. The EEG graph, however, would show that blood pressure, respiration, pulse rate, and temperature were all on the descent. The brain-wave recording no longer traces smooth alpha rhythms, but a small, constantly changing pattern.

In this stage the mind begins to wander over events of the day that require no great concentration . . . the memory of having run into a friend or having bought a pair of shoes. During this prelude to deep sleep, the mere mention of a person's name wakes him up.

As he drifts into stage two, he is no longer able to see, even if he is one of those rare people who sleeps with his eyes open. Slowly his eyeballs move from side to side, while the amplitude and frequency of the brain waves increase. Mental images which bear little relation to each other may flash through the mind: One minute he is thinking about his grandmother's funeral, the next about an argument he had with his boss. Although it is not difficult to rouse a person from stage two sleep, he continues this way for twenty to thirty minutes if undisturbed.

At stage three, delta waves begin to emerge as the characteristic pattern. Temperature and blood pressure drop even further and the sleeper is almost completely relaxed. This is the time when restless sleepers do their tossing and turning and talkers do their muttering. People do dream at this stage, but usually they don't remember it when shaken awake. Stage two dreamers are easy to rouse, however, and can often recall a dream in vivid detail.

Continuing the descent into the unconscious, the sleeper finally reaches stage four, or delta sleep, when large, slow delta waves roll regularly across the EEG screen. Delta sleep, which lasts about twenty minutes, represents total relaxation and loss of conscious control; this is the time when people wet their beds and walk in their sleep.

Until recently it was thought that the sleeper plunged from a state of wakefulness to unconsciousness, rising up in the morning like a phoenix from the ashes. It turns out that the situation is more complicated. A night's sleep actually consists of four or five cycles of a rise from stage four up to stage two, then a return down to stage four. Although the average complete sleep cycle takes roughly an hour and a half, individuals may vary considerably according to their own built-in time clocks.

The later stage two phases are not the same as the first one. In the later phases, it will take a loud noise to open a person's eyes, not merely the mention of his name. Whereas the eyeballs moved slowly on the first trip into stage two, they now move very rapidly: Thus the name REM (Rapid Eye Movement) sleep for this phase. The body is totally relaxed—in fact, the chin may be drooping and the mouth open. Nevertheless, the brain-wave pattern is very similar to the pattern of someone who is fully awake.

During each period of sleep, people have many dreams, the majority of which have fled from memory before the next morning. Most remembered dreaming takes place in the last REM cycle before waking up.

Consequences of sleep deprivation

The importance of REM sleep was first demonstrated by Dr. William Dement of Stanford University in the early 1960s. Each time a study volunteer slid into the REM phase, Dr. Dement awakened him with a buzzer. As the experiment continued through several nights, subjects became increasingly hard to arouse—their bodies seemed to be fighting deprivation of REM sleep, although they were getting plenty of stages three and four sleep. The morning afterwards they tended to be short-tempered and touchy.

When Dr. Dement allowed these brave souls to sleep through an entire night undisturbed, he discovered a curious fact: REM sleep predominated, as it did for the next several nights, until the subject appeared to have caught up with his lost REM time.

The importance of the other extreme—deep sleep—was demonstrated by another researcher, Dr. Wilse B. Webb of the University of Florida. Her subjects were allowed to drift through stages two and three, but a soft buzzer prevented them from reaching stage four, although the sound did not wake them up. The following day everyone plodded along at a slow pace, and many felt morose and ill-equipped to face the world. When allowed to return to normal sleep, they spent several nights catching up on lost deep sleep.

Of course some people are forced, through the nature of their jobs, to go for long periods with no sleep. Doctors work three-day shifts at the hospital, grabbing only a nap here and there. A young man with a large family tries to make ends meet by holding down two jobs or by working many hours of overtime. Tireless folks sail through holiday seasons with barely a wink between festivities.

Although most people snap back to normal after a night or two, studies hint that sleep loss stretching over a period of time may have damaging effects on the brain. Further, as one might expect, the older the person, the less able he is to tolerate prolonged sleep loss.

A study carried out by an army psychologist revealed that sleep loss not only slows down people's reaction time and impairs judgment, it also makes their reactions erratic and unpredictable. Of a group of soldiers deprived of sleep for thirty hours, many showed a peculiar variation in their ability to react from one minute to the next. For example, one minute the subject might easily catch a ball thrown his way; five minutes later, a two-second lag in reaction time would cause him to fumble.

Some people sleep too much

Some people, whether from boredom, emotional upset, or "laziness," fall into the habit of deliberately drifting back to sleep even when they are quite ready to get up. Certainly, sleep is a pleasure for most people, but consistent oversleeping can have as adverse an effect on performance of the day's duties as sleeping too little. Oversleepers often feel sluggish for the entire day, because their basal metabolism has dropped so low.

A survey by the American Cancer Society reveals that people who consistently sleep more than ten hours a night have twice as many heart attacks and three and a half times as many fatal strokes as those who sleep seven hours or less. The survey did not indicate whether the long sleepers had been that way all their lives or were recent converts; thus no definite conclusions can be drawn.

Certainly, many people spend more time than they need to in bed simply because they do not like the prospect of getting up to face what lies ahead. A senior partner in a public-accounting firm found himself in this situation when his office was reorganized and he was given a less interesting job. He knew that the firm had fallen on hard times, that a few people were in line for being fired, and others would be squeezed out one way or another. He suspected that he might not survive the purge.

Although this man had always prided himself on catching the

7:42 suburban train no matter how little sleep he had had or how much work lay on his desk, suddenly he found himself unable to respond to the alarm clock or to the worried urging of his wife. He would pull the blankets over his head and sink back for another thirty minutes or so, by which time he had missed two trains. Weekends he would loll around till nine or ten o'clock, by which time he had missed a golf match.

Unconsciously, perhaps, he was hastening the blow which he knew was coming. Eventually he was fired. Several months later he realized what his new-found sleep habits had cost him in a firm that valued punctuality above all other virtues. When he landed a better job in another city, all of his former punctiliousness returned, the lawn was mowed on Saturday morning, and the Sunday golfing partners were not disappointed.

How sleep patterns develop

As everyone knows, babies require a lot more sleep than their parents. A newborn will clock some sixteen to eighteen hours per day in the crib, while his father sleeps seven or eight hours and his grandfather only six or seven hours. Also, while the baby spends about half his time in delta sleep, the figure is more like 20 per cent for Dad and almost zero for Granddad.

All three are subject to the circadian rhythm that rules all living things—the built-in timing device that is synchronized with the daily 24-hour turn of the earth. Because of this circadian rhythm, a man from Boston will wake up at 4 A.M. on his first morning in Seattle, instead of his customary 7 A.M.

In primitive societies, everybody sleeps at night and does his active business during the day. The forces of civilization have tended to distort the circadian rhythm, however, so that some people feel most alive and awake at night, while others are ready to fall asleep at 8 P.M. Modern technology has made it easier for night owls: Lights shine in the streets from dusk till dawn and taxis run all night. In primitive societies there is not much to do at night except go to bed.

While periods of sleep correspond naturally with periods of darkness, Richard Deming in *Sleep, Our Unknown Life* notes with interest that Arctic Circle dwellers keep essentially the same schedule through the constant darkness of winter as through the daylight summer, although in winter they sleep about an hour longer.

Many night owls fool people into believing that they get by on virtually no sleep, since they always seem to be up when phoned. In truth, these people may be addicted to catnapping, a habit common in older people. Often a few minutes of dozing in the early evening —leaning back in a chair rather than stretched out full-length on a bed—renews mind and body for the evening ahead. Winston Churchill, a dedicated catnapper even in his youth, claimed that the practice could turn one day into two for him.

If you have time, a full-fledged nap may provide more strength for the long haul than merely a few minutes of dozing. Physical-fitness addict Senator William Proxmire of Wisconsin frequently sneaks in a half-hour nap on his office couch, a habit he learned from his physician father. This practice, he maintains, can be a great boon to people who work long hours under pressure. At least three recent presidents—Truman, Kennedy, and Johnson—took regular naps in the middle of the day.

For the majority of us, a night of unbroken sleep is the most practical approach to health. Experiments have shown that normal sleepers subjected to several interruptions during the night are much less sharp the following day—as any mother of a newborn can confirm.

As a final word of encouragement for the confirmed night owl, here are some possible techniques for bringing your time schedule into line with the rest of the world's:

• Don't let yourself sleep too long. If you can determine your ideal sleeping time and stick to the schedule, you will have a better chance of waking up spontaneously with a cheerful attitude toward the day ahead. A good time to determine the ideal sleeping span is on a vacation; go to bed when you are tired and get up when you're ready, not when the clock says you should.

• Keep to a regular schedule so that your body has a chance to develop strong internal rhythms.

• Get out of bed gradually rather than bounding up and staggering to the bathroom. Stretch your limbs, wiggle your toes, sit up slowly and put your feet on the floor. Limber your shoulders by hunching them high, then letting them sag. Count to five in each position and repeat four times. Stand up and stretch your arms high for a count of ten, then bend over and try touching your toes, letting the knees flex. Do this several times.

The point of all this limbering up is to get the bloodstream flowing, lungs pumping, and brain synapses snapping right away instead of at noon, your normal time for feeling more than half alive.

• Try to develop a positive attitude toward getting up in the morning by making it a more pleasant experience. For instance, set the alarm for fifteen minutes earlier and read your favorite part of the newspaper in bed along with a cup of coffee. Once you have accumulated a few good memories of morning experiences, the prospect of waking up will be more pleasant.

Fighting insomnia

Not only is insomnia a very common source of distress; it is extremely difficult to treat, because its causes are so numerous.

As Dr. Ernest Hartmann points out, the doctor's job would be much easier if he had a few ready labels for different types of insomnia. "At the moment it must be considered a final common pathway—a symptom of a great many different processes."

Dr. Hartmann asks himself the following question: Does the patient have trouble falling asleep, or staying asleep? Usually, unless a person is sick or depressed, his insomnia is of the falling-asleep variety. Often he is tense and afraid of the "letting go" that follows loss of consciousness. Such people are much more easily treated than those whose insomnia is of the waking-up variety.

Here is Dr. Hartmann's list of the common causes for the two types of insomnia he identifies:

Difficulty in Falling Asleep

• Pain of any medical origin, often not noticed during the day but causing discomfort at bedtime; for example, poison ivy itches more and menstrual cramps are more severe at night when one is lying in bed;

• Nonspecific stress and anxiety—for instance, anticipation of a busy day which will include firing an employee, buying one's wife a birthday present, phoning the broker about a stock that is plunging, and returning a warped fishing rod;

• Specific fears and anxieties, especially those relating to "letting go" or losing control. The insomniac may find his road to sleep blocked by fear of dying, or by worry that sexual or aggressive impulses will emerge in his dreams;

• A heavy, late meal which has not had time to digest.

Difficulty in Remaining Asleep
(Night or Early Morning Awakenings)

• Medical conditions which get worse during the night: epilepsy, angina, peptic ulcer, asthma;

• Rare neurological disease involving the hypothalamus or the brain stem;

• Hypothyroidism or other endocrine abnormalities;

• Anticipation of an exciting event;

• Depression. In certain kinds of depression, awakenings during the night or early morning may be the only indication of the person's psychological condition (see Chapter 13).

Whatever the cause of insomnia, the phenomenon is widespread. According to one set of figures, half the American population suffers from insomnia at least occasionally, and there may be as many as thirty million chronic sufferers. Americans shell out half a billion dollars for sedatives and tranquilizers every year, and no one knows how many bottles of alcohol are consumed as sleep-inducing measures.

There is a booming market for mechanical sleep aids, from eye blinders and earplugs to vibrating beds. Many insomniacs have invested money in the water bed which appeared on the market a few years ago, with varying reports of success. Other sufferers are constantly on the lookout for "natural" methods of going to sleep, such as taking a steam bath or doing yoga exercises.

Predictably, a vast arsenal of folk remedies has been applied to the age-old problem of insomnia. Some are pure nonsense and depend for effectiveness on the power of suggestion. Others have a sound medical basis.

For example, many people find that drinking a glass of warm milk before bed, as Grandmother prescribed, helps lull them to sleep. Scientists have discovered that milk contains an amino acid called tryptophan, which in concentrated form has a strong sedative effect.

In addition, milk revives memories of the soothing days spent at Mother's breast.

Modern approaches

In the nineteenth century, even intelligent people believed that it was important to sleep with one's head pointing north, in order to take advantage of the sleep-inducing electrical current that ran from the North to the South Pole. Although of course there is no such current, it is true—as the Russians discovered in the 1950s—that an electric current will help induce sleep.

The electrosleep machine which they devised sends gentle waves through the brain of the patient, who is attached to the machine. The half-hour treatment produces a feeling of relaxation and a sense of well-being, and the Russians claim great success with it. Americans have been more skeptical, although so far they have not been able to point to any harmful side effects. The treatment does not work for everybody, but it has brought about some dramatic cures.

Presently there are only three clinics in the United States whose main purpose is to treat the chronic insomniac rather than merely carry out sleep experiments: one at Dartmouth Medical School, one at the Medical School in Hershey, Pennsylvania, and the largest at Stanford University School of Medicine, Palo Alto, California. At these institutions, patients undergo extensive testing to determine whether the insomnia is neurological in origin, secondary to a medical or psychological problem, or genetic. When all data are analyzed, recommendations for therapy are discussed.

Dr. Peter Hauri, Director of the Dartmouth Sleep Laboratory, estimates that at least three out of four patients can expect dramatic improvement in their ability to sleep. He also points out that some patients who come to him are worrying unnecessarily about eccentric sleep habits. One engineer who sought treatment at his wife's urging had been averaging only four hours of sleep nightly for his entire life. Testing revealed that the man merely had a remarkable ability to drop quickly into deep delta sleep, then come directly up to the REM stage. He really didn't need more than four hours of sleep.

A thirty-five-year-old housewife appeared in the lab with the opposite problem: She just didn't feel right without thirteen hours of sleep. Unable to find anything wrong with her, Dr. Hauri concluded that the thirteen hours was what that woman needed.

"The main thing is not to exaggerate the importance of losing a night's sleep," he urges. "It might make a person feel bad but, as a number of studies have shown, it will have practically no effect upon his objective efficiency. It would take three or four nights of no sleep at all before his ability to perform actually went down."

Possible physiological explanations for inability to fall asleep are numerous. For instance, a person may have trouble metabolizing serotonin, the brain chemical thought to be related to sleep. Or he may be unable to produce serotonin from its precursor, tryptophane, which is found in various protein foods, including milk. And not to overlook the obvious, he may be drinking coffee, tea, or some other stimulating beverage too late at night.

Dr. Hauri claims that sleep clinics "cure" about as successfully as any physician or psychiatrist. Some patients get dramatically better; the majority show at least some improvement and leave therapy much happier. The one patient in four who finds no help at the sleep clinic is often relieved simply to know more about his condition, which he is now able to perceive as less than catastrophic.

One consistent laboratory revelation is that the person who claims "I didn't sleep a wink all night" actually did drop off for several hours, although he was not in the deeper stages of sleep. The insomniac may feel like he has been awake all night and may honestly believe it, but it seldom is the case.

Bedtime rituals

Many people go through elaborate preparations for bed every night, although they may not be aware of it. One young lady was absolutely unable to fall asleep without a glass of water next to her bed, fearing that she might get thirsty during the night (which seldom happened). She also kept a Kleenex firmly clenched in her right hand, in case she needed to blow her nose.

The smoker is often unable to sleep without a final cigarette, which may in fact disturb his breathing during the night. The food addict cannot turn off the lights without a last bite of something. If the something is not very light, such as a cup of soup, he may find himself sleeping poorly and waking up at 3 A.M. in the midst of a nightmare.

The alcoholic may claim that a final hypnotic dose of scotch is just what he needs to guarantee a good night's sleep. Alcohol, however, has a disruptive effect on recorded sleep, and the insomniac who is a heavy drinker will often find that sleep comes much easier without it (see Chapter 7).

The mayor of a western city claims he is utterly unable to sleep unless his shoes are placed side by side under the bed. He discovered this peculiarity one night when his wife moved them to the closet. She herself will fret and worry unless all the dishes have been taken out of the dishwasher.

Omission of a part of our little rituals can make a temporary insomniac out of any of us. While the first instinct may be to reach for the bottle of sleeping pills in the medicine chest, it is always wiser to consider other possibilities first—among them, whether one is the victim of an unrecognized bedtime compulsion.

Dr. Hartmann urges physicians to use caution when prescribing sleeping pills and to do as careful a medical and psychological workup as possible beforehand. Naturally, if the patient has an illness, he must be treated. But in many cases of insomnia, psychological support and some practical hints can go a long way toward providing relief.

Other hints for the temporary insomniac

For the mild insomniac who is only slightly depressed or anxious and for whom psychotherapy is unnecessary, undesirable, or too expensive, several bits of information could prove helpful:

• Some people who lead irregular lives will find that their insomnia is relieved by the institution of a regular daily schedule, including eating at specific hours and going to bed at the same time each night.

• Mild exercise at least two hours before going to bed is often effective in lulling the body to rest. But don't start jumping rope ten minutes before bedtime; you may find yourself too charged up to fall asleep immediately.

• It is difficult to predict the effects of different foods on different people. Ulcer specialists, for instance, are locked in debate over whether bland diets really do anything for the ulcer sufferer. Some people, however, know from their own experience that sharp and spicy foods upset their stomachs; thus they should avoid them before bedtime.

On the other hand, foods with a great deal of roughage such as carrots, lettuce and celery, may conspire to produce increased intestinal activity, which also inhibits a peaceful night's rest.

Final notes on sleep research

Although researchers have contributed much to our knowledge of the physiology and chemistry of sleep, no one yet has found the answer to the basic question: Why is it that we need sleep? Throughout the centuries man has proclaimed the virtues of a good night's rest, but we still do not know how the restorative effects are achieved.

One thing experimenters have learned: Sleep is not a wasted period when the brain is lying idle rather than taking in new information. Several years ago records which taught a foreign language while the listener was asleep were popular. Many scientists were skeptical of the advertised benefits, pointing out that the brain needs sleep as much as the body and that interfering with normal brain activity could lead to problems.

Nobody ever came across with solid evidence of the evils wrought by sleep learning, but the technique never really caught on. Instinctively, it would appear, people strive to protect their sleeping life as much as their waking one from intrusion by unknown forces.

Sleep philosophers line up roughly in two camps: those who believe that the restorative processes are begun during the sleeping hours, when brain tissue is resynthesized, and those who feel that sleep is a state of being to which we have been conditioned for survival.

The latter argument holds that cave men would have been wasting a lot of energy hunting for food at night, when they couldn't see and when various predatory animals were roaming around. Therefore, it is theorized, they had to learn to do something else with their time.

One interesting observation has been made about animals: Creatures susceptible to attack, such as rabbits and deer, sleep very little and lightly, while lions may snore their way through sixteen hours of the day. In other words, there are curious and unexplained ties between the needs of a species for sleep and for safety. Predators can afford to relax; the weaker animals must stay on their guard.

BIBLIOGRAPHY

Deming, Richard. *Sleep, Our Unknown Life*. Nelson, 1972.

Hartmann, Ernest, M.D. "How to Help Your Patients Sleep Better," *Medical Times,* Mar. 1972, vol. 100, no. 3.

————. "Psychological Differences Between Long and Short Sleepers," *Archives of General Psychiatry,* May 1972, vol. 26.

Proxmire, William. "Everybody Sleep!" *Family Health,* Oct. 1973.

Scarf, Maggie. "Oh, for a Decent Night's Sleep!" *New York Times Magazine,* Oct. 21, 1973.

Segal, Julius, M.D. "How Much Sleep Do You Need?" *U.S. News & World Report,* Dec. 28, 1970.

Young, Warren R. "Five Rules for Waking Up Alert," *Reader's Digest,* June 1972.

4 NOISE IS TIRING

One urban aggravation which is only now coming to be identified as the perpetrator of a number of crimes, including fatigue, is noise pollution.

A century ago physicians were aware that blacksmiths, boilermakers, and others who worked amidst constant banging and clanging often became deaf after a few years. Today, in a world noisier than ever, scientists are constantly uncovering evidence of the relationship of noise not only to hearing loss, but to nervous disorders, irritability, inefficiency, and fatigue.

All of us are threatened by noise pollution some of the time, and some of us all of the time. Of course, a world without sound would be a dangerous place. Without the rumble of an approaching truck, we might step out into the street; without the whirr of an electric fan, a child might stick his fingers between the blades.

In recent times, however, the usefulness of noise has given way more and more to its disturbing properties. Heavy garbage trucks clang through the streets; construction workers drill relentlessly into the pavement; planes boom overhead; lawn mowers shatter the calm of a Saturday morning.

In our offices, typewriters provide a staccato background for our working hours, while out in the streets, blaring transistor radios add to the clamor of traffic. And the lifeless strains of canned music pursue us relentlessly into restaurants, elevators, and department stores.

How much noise is too much? Sound is measured in decibels, one decibel representing the smallest difference of loudness that the normal human ear can detect between two sounds. Conversation in a relatively quiet setting measures about 60 decibels, while the roar of traffic or the noise of a machine shop reaches up to 80. Any sound higher than 80 is likely to make us uncomfortable; sustained sounds of more than 90 decibels can be dangerous to mental and physical health.

Sounds which reach the danger level: a jet plane taking off, 150 decibels; a subway train screeching along the track, 95; a power lawn mower, 96; a newspaper printing press, 97; a food blender, 85.

Doctors have discovered that noise pollution is as much a threat to certain susceptible people as air pollution to people with emphysema or asthma. Several studies indicate that either prolonged exposure to noise or sudden, sharp noise will produce involuntary responses by the vascular, digestive, and nervous systems. The danger to the cilia of the inner ear is obvious, but the more subtle physiologic and emotional responses are not yet fully known.

If someone bangs a pair of cymbals next to your ear, your body responds in the same way as if someone were pointing a gun at you: Epinephrine shoots into the blood, the heart beats rapidly, the blood vessels constrict, the pupils dilate, the head turns, the skin pales, and the stomach, esophagus, and intestines are seized by spasms. When the noise is prolonged, the heart begins to flutter. In animal experiments, rabbits subjected to eight weeks of extreme noise showed elevated cholesterol levels as well as increased constriction of the aorta.

Extensive studies of both animals and humans have also established that prolonged exposure to high-decibel noise, such as residents of a jetport town endure, results in definite hearing loss. Even the residents of a large city will find their hearing eventually less sharp than that of their country cousins.

Also, psychiatrists believe that people who are exposed to prolonged noise are more easily affected by disturbances. They are more inclined to fly into a rage or to launch an argument on slight provocation.

"Perhaps the most important aspect of noise is its effect on the quality of life," an official of the Environmental Protection Agency points out. "The interruption of sleep and conversation, the strain of having to shout and listen over the roar of air compressors and the pounding of jackhammers, are just isolated examples of the indignities caused by noise. Especially unnecessary noise, which seems to be particularly provoking and has been blamed for triggering murder, suicide, and insanity.

"Less dramatic but certainly prevalent are the cases of sudden loss of temper, child abuse, headache, sleeplessness, depression, and irritability caused by the intrusion of noise into our private lives."

Recently a California otolaryngologist, Dr. Maurice Schiff, reported that noise severely disturbs both the quality and duration of sleep. While the roar of the early-morning truck traffic might not be enough to bring a city dweller to his feet, it can seriously inhibit the critical REM (rapid eye movement) stage of his sleep cycle, when dreaming takes place. People who are deprived of their REM sleep are usually tired, irritable, and distracted the next day.

Further, Dr. Schiff explains, an environment where sudden, irregular, or inappropriate sounds are common can bring on an emotional crisis in a person already on the edge. Other studies indicate that unrelenting noise can make us introverted, uninterested in sex, and clumsy in the performance of complicated tasks.

The pessimistic German philosopher Arthur Schopenhauer maintained that people who are not sensitive to noise are likewise indifferent to "argument, or thought, or poetry, or art, in a word, to any kind of intellectual influence." Many great writers have claimed an aversion to noise, which interrupts concentration. Schopenhauer was particularly irritated by the cracking of whips.

"Occasionally it happens that some slight but constant noise continues to bother and distract me for a time before I become distinctly conscious of it," he commented. "All I feel is a steady increase in the labor of thinking—just as though I were trying to walk with a weight on my foot. At last I find out what it is."

What is the solution?

Legislation for noise control is minimal at both state and national levels, although various citizens' groups have been able to bring about control of local situations: limiting the noise levels at construction sites, rerouting low-flying jets, for example.

A major reason for the lack of public pressure for antinoise laws is that a lot of people seem to find noise reassuring. A few years ago Ray Donley, a New Jersey acoustical engineer, told an American Medical Association symposium on environmental health that "in many cases, a quiet piece of equipment won't sell. Detroit spends thousands of dollars to create just the right sound for slamming car doors," he reports.

"And a nearly silent vacuum cleaner—which is technically feasible—is not likely to sell very well. Unless it sounds powerful, today's woman won't believe it is really cleaning."

For people who long for a peaceful environment, the ideal solution might be to pack up for a place where there is no unnecessary noise. Such places are becoming harder and harder to find. Maine, for instance, was once considered the ultimate in bucolic tranquility. Now the winter peace is shattered by the roar of snowmobiles.

As a desperate antidote to the current state of affairs, many Americans have taken to wearing earplugs at night and even during the day. Others attempt to soundproof their houses or apartments with padded carpets, heavy drapes, or wall corking. Some people have even tried hypnotism.

At the moment, all contractors doing business with the government are limited to a decibel level of 90. Until tougher regulations are put into effect for other noisemakers, the fatigue sufferer who counts noise as a major problem can do little but write his congressman or form his own citizens group.

In Chicago, the Citizens Against Noise organization has called for a Think Quiet movement, on the premise that the best way to combat noise pollution is to prevent it. In Memphis, "Silent Citizen" awards are given to residents who perform such civil acts as putting mufflers on their lawn mowers. Police in that city arrest more than a thousand horn honkers each year.

But before casting stones at others, it might be wise to check whether you yourself are making unnecessary noise. Here are a few reminders:

• Walk across the floor, don't stomp. Spare the neighbors underneath, and your own family.

• Don't shout when you're mad.

• Slip out of your shoes, don't drop them on the floor.

• Use plastic garbage cans.

• Put carpets on the floors.

• Keep the radio, TV or stereo at a level high enough to hear, not louder.

• Check out decibel levels of appliances before purchase.

• Train a dog not to bark every time a door opens.

• Don't walk around in public places carrying a transistor radio.

• Don't sit on a motorcycle and race the motor.

• Don't honk your car horn except in emergencies.

• Don't slam doors.

BIBLIOGRAPHY

Aronson, Harvey. "Noise Noise Noise!" *Cosmopolitan,* May 1972.

"How Today's Noise Hurts Body and Mind," *Medical World News,* June 13, 1969.

Navarra, John Gabriel. *Our Noisy World.* Doubleday, 1969.

"Quiet, Please!" *Newsweek,* Dec. 17, 1973.

Schopenhauer, Arthur. "On Noise," translated by T. Bailey Saunders, *Great Essays,* ed. Houston Peterson. Washington Square Press, 1953.

5 EXERCISE KEEPS YOU YOUNG

"How can you talk about getting more exercise when I'm so tired most of the time I can barely brush my teeth in the morning?" Ray queried his doctor. At the age of forty-two, Ray is fairly close to his ideal weight and in good health. The demands of job and family, however, leave him little time for relaxation. Weekends are generally spent making minor repairs on the house or making pilgrimages to his wife's invalid mother.

"Why don't you just try walking to the train station, Ray, instead of having your wife drive you?" his physician suggested. "And walk home too, no matter how steep that hill looks at 6 P.M. Just try it for a week."

Ray tried, and now he swears he'll never set foot in the car again, even if it means missing a train. The forty-five minutes of walking each day has lightened his outlook on life and recharged his batteries.

The sense of well-being that exercise produces has both a physiological and a psychological basis. First, during exercise the circulation of blood to the brain increases, making you feel more alive. Second, exercise is fun, or at least it should be. It lifts the cloud of boredom and takes the edge off tension.

When Ray walks to the train station, he drinks in the surroundings, inhales the odors of fresh cut grass and flowering trees, feels the warmth of the summer air on his skin. In winter he exults in the bite of the cold air and looks forward to a cup of coffee at the station house.

As Dr. Paul Dudley White expressed it, "Mental and spiritual fitness, both dependent on a good brain, are greatly enhanced by optimal physical fitness. Body, mind, and soul are inextricably woven together, and whatever helps or hurts any one of these three sides of the whole man helps or hurts the other two. We need for our brain the purest blood possible, uncontaminated by nicotine or other poisons, and in ample quantity supplied by a healthy circulation."

Dr. White, for many years the best-known heart specialist in this country, was a familiar sight on his bicycle, and he was also a dedicated walker. His strong convictions about exercise were based on "my deep feeling of the importance of the use of leg muscles as an integral part of the maintenance of a proper circulation.

"Studies have shown—and this may come as somewhat of a surprise—that when a person is walking, about 30 per cent of the circulation of the blood is carried on by the leg muscles, and the remaining per cent by the heart."

When we use our legs, blood is pushed upward—against the law of gravity—through the body into the heart. This spares the overburdened heart and, in Dr. White's opinion, considerably reduces the chance of heart attack.

Vigorous use of the leg muscles also tends to prevent the blood from clotting and keeps the veins clear of clots. Many illnesses today are caused by the tendency of the blood to coagulate; in the arteries of the heart, causing thrombosis, in the brain vessels, causing strokes, and in the leg veins, causing pulmonary embolism.

"Still another reason for the use of the leg muscles is that the fatigue produced by it is undoubtedly the best tranquilizer ever made, either by nature or by man," Dr. White pointed out.

His sentiments are echoed by many doctors, particularly cardiologists, whose business it is to observe the effects of exercise on health. Dr. Theodore L. Klumpp, a member of the AMA's Committee on Aging, makes this comment: "Continued physical activity often makes the difference between a fine figure of a man at age seventy, and a man burdened by aches and pains and boredom—if, indeed, the chair-bound man lives to age seventy."

People who enjoy sports can remember the exhilaration of running down a hockey field or around a baseball diamond during school days; the joy of mastering a particular skill, the heightened sense of aliveness that came from using one's body. Even non-sports enthusiasts might have enjoyed being out of doors.

Why, then, does interest wane as the years slip by? How does the star high-school basketball player wind up doing nothing more athletic than running down the front steps and stooping to pick up the newspaper?

First, there are the obvious problems of logistics. Much as one might like to jump into a good game of volleyball, it is not always possible to get to the local YMCA, nor is it easy to collect a team from among the neighbors.

Another reason is the irrational but common fear that physical activity is harmful for people who have reached middle age. Although nobody would recommend that a person with a heart condition start rowing for two hours a day, there is a form of exercise suitable for each person. One thinks of President Harry Truman and his famous morning walks, which he continued almost until his death.

Labor-saving devices have also contributed heavily to the national laziness; today we can get by with a minimum of movement. Remote control even eliminates the necessity of getting off the sofa to change the TV channel.

"As man grows lazier, he grows fatter—his heart, his arteries, his muscles, his glands degenerate," Dr. Klumpp warns. "The extra time that machines have provided us should be spent not in sedentary pursuits such as watching TV, but in physical activity."

Another factor in the decline of exercise which Dr. Klumpp considers important: delusions of status. "As a man moves up the ladder of success, he begins to feel that it is unbecoming to get out and make minor repairs on the house or wash and polish the car. Shouldn't one who has made the grade leave such work to others? False pride keeps many men and women from doing work they would really like to do."

Advice from the experts

Walking is the cheapest, easiest, and most accessible form of exercise, and it can be done by people of any age and at any time of day. Dr. White suggests walking at a pace of three to four miles per hour for at least one hour every day, or seven hours per week if a daily stretch is not possible. Brisk walking is a fine conditioner because it brings nearly every muscle into play.

Since the main point is to get your legs moving, many activities —tennis, golf (without a cart), swimming, skiing, gardening, mountain climbing, dancing (but not during or right after dinner)—also serve the purpose well. Jogging should be undertaken only after checking first with a physician, unless one is unquestionably young and healthy.

People who honestly don't have the time or the interest to pursue a sport should make a double effort to step up routine daily activities: for example, climb stairs instead of taking the elevator, park the car a mile from the office and walk to work.

One hundred years ago, when America was a farm society, no one had to worry about getting enough exercise. Unfortunately, we cannot all head back to the farm and become laborers, so we must compromise. As Dr. White observed, "Man is not yet all brain. We must recognize this fact and do what we can to use our muscles as nature intended."

Of course, the more vigorous the exercise, the better; however, any activity that puts muscles into action and takes the mind off problems is beneficial. Muscles that aren't used become flabby, sluggish, and less capable of moving into action when needed.

"The main thing is to find something that is fun to do," Dr. Klumpp advises. "Most of us secretly yearn to take part in some sport—it's an extension of our play instinct. But we hold off. We're too ashamed or too clumsy or too embarrassed. My advice is to keep two things in mind: No one ever starts an expert, and it doesn't really matter whether you win or lose. What counts is the fun, the friendship, the movement."

Many people carry in the back of their minds stories of men who have dropped dead on the golf course or the tennis courts with no warning and with no previous history of illness. The connection between death and athletic activity is merely circumstantial, however. Actually, such attacks are the result of a long and gradual process of degeneration of the arteries. Studies show that almost 50 per cent of all heart attacks occur during sleep; when they don't, the finger of accusation is usually pointed at whatever the victim was doing at the time.

What about exercise machines that do half the work for you? Dr. Klumpp acknowledges that they are better than nothing, but stresses that "one of the great benefits you get from exercise on your own, especially in sports, is that it's play, it's fun, a boon to good mental health. Exercise isn't just a matter of muscular activity. It steps up all the body's functions, improves posture, helps you get rid of pent-up anxieties and frustrations."

Women need exercise too

When doctors speak of the need to stay in good health through a daily exercise program, it is usually men they are thinking of. After all, the reasoning goes, women live longer and are less prone to coronary disease. For them, exercise is chiefly a means to weight control.

Not true: Lack of exercise can create severe problems for women as well as men. Some years ago, for example, Dr. Evalyn S. Gendel, director of the division of maternal and child health, Kansas State Department of Health, studied one hundred women aged eighteen to twenty-three who complained of chronic low backache and fatigue following pregnancy.

After eliminating orthopedic, pelvic, renal, and psychological causes, she was left with thirty-five patients, all of whom had the following characteristics: a history of irregular physical activity since childhood, poorly developed anterior abdominal muscles, and a variety of other post-delivery complaints which affected their ability to function. When these women were put on a program of gradual physical conditioning, symptoms disappeared in as few as six months.

Although the study was a small one, Dr. Gendel feels that it illustrates a little-recognized problem in this country. "The general public, the educational system, and medical science have been largely indifferent to the general physical fitness or performance of the non-athletic woman, the 'ordinary female' in the population," she observes.

Although efforts toward change are being made, old attitudes linger on. For instance, both men and women are still influenced by the old myths about athletic women being "too masculine" or about "biological differences" between the sexes. There is no scientific evidence supporting the contention that women by nature are less fitted for exercise and competition.

Working off unwanted pounds

The equation for weight control is a simple one: Consume the same number of calories that you burn off. Extra calories provide unneeded energy which is stored as fat on the body.

The number of calories your body requires depends on age, body build, and other factors. The average man will burn 2,400 to 4,500 calories per day, depending on the amount and kind of exercise he is getting. Athletes may put away as many as 6,000 calories per day and not gain weight.

The American Medical Association points out that people have labored for years under two misconceptions about exercise: first, that a great deal of it is necessary before weight can be materially affected; and second, that exercise increases the appetite. Experiments on both men and animals have demonstrated that both these assumptions are false.

First, study the chart below.

Energy Expenditure by a 150-pound Person in Various Activities*

Activity	Gross Energy Cost-Cal per hr.
A. Rest and Light Activity 50–200	
Lying down or sleeping 80	
Sitting 100	
Driving an automobile 120	
Standing 140	
Domestic work 180	

Activity	Gross Energy Cost-Cal per hr.

B. Moderate Activity 200–350
Bicycling (5½ mph) 210
Walking (2½ mph) 210
Gardening 220
Canoeing (2½ mph) 230
Golf 250
Lawn mowing (power mower) 250
Bowling 270
Lawn mowing (hand mower) 270
Fencing 300
Rowboating (2½ mph) 300
Swimming (¼ mph) 300
Walking (3¾ mph) 300
Badminton 350
Horseback riding (trotting) 350
Square dancing 350
Volleyball 350
Roller skating 350

C. Vigorous Activity ....over 350
Table tennis 360
Ditch digging (hand shovel) 400
Ice skating (10 mph) 400
Wood chopping or sawing 400
Tennis 420
Water skiing 480
Hill climbing (100 ft. per hr.) 490
Skiing (10 mph) 600
Squash and handball 600
Cycling (13 mph) 660
Scull rowing (race) 840
Running (10 mph) 900

Prepared by Robert E. Johnson, M.D., Ph.D., and colleagues, Department of Physiology and Biophysics, University of Illinois, August, 1967.
* The standards represent a compromise between those proposed by the British Medical Association (1950), Christensen (1953) and Wells, Balke, and Van Fossan (1956). Where available, actual measured values have been used; for other values a "best guess" was made.

The figures on energy expenditure are probably underestimates, because of the way they were arrived at: The amount of oxygen consumed during a specific exercise period was compared with the equivalent number of calories burned. In fact, what happens is that the effects of exercise continue after the actual time during which a person is exerting himself. Body metabolism has been stepped up, and it returns to normal only gradually. This process requires energy.

Of course, the number of calories burned will vary according to how vigorously a sport is being performed and how much the performer weighs. A teen-ager weighing 100 pounds will burn as few as 50 calories walking 15 minutes at 3 mph, while her 200-pound father will use up as many as 80 calories in the same length of time and at the same pace.

It is true that you cannot burn off weight overnight, no matter how hard you exercise. It is also true that although you must walk thirty-five miles to lose a pound of fat, you don't have to make the whole trip at once. You can also lose ten pounds in a year by walking an extra mile a day, as long as your eating habits remain the same.

Unfortunately, studies have shown that while we grow older and fatter, our appetites do not diminish. In other words, a high-school graduate who takes an office job tends to exercise less, but continues out of habit to eat as much as ever.

Help for the aching back

Low back pain has reached almost endemic proportions in twentieth-century America. It is estimated that seven million people are under treatment of some kind for an aching back, the ailment which ranks as the top drain on industrial-compensation funds.

Perhaps the most famous back-pain victims in recent times are President John F. Kennedy, who suffered for twenty-five years as a result of a war injury, and his brother, Senator Edward Kennedy, whose back was wrenched in a plane crash. In their cases, the pain was the obvious result of direct physical injury. For most people, there is no clear-cut triggering factor. Although it is assumed that "back trouble" can run in a family, no clearly defined hereditary mechanism exists.

Recently, researchers have come to the conclusion that probably the most important predisposing factor to back trouble is lack of exercise, combined with stress. Many people spend a quarter of their lives sitting at a desk or a typewriter, under the stress and strain of a competitive office situation which causes them to tense up. When muscles remain contracted for long periods, special measures are needed to relax them.

The modern car is another backache-producer. It keeps people from walking, and it condemns them to the worst possible sitting posture (the "better" the car, the more likely you are to be slumped low in an overstuffed seat with no support for the small of your back).

The path to low back pain is well-recognized in several instances. Obese people often suffer from it, as do pregnant women. Enlargement of the prostate may lead to low back pain in men. Other causes include tumors, arthritis, rheumatism, and infections. Emotional factors, including tension, anxiety, and depression, have been implicated by some estimates in as many as 80 per cent of cases.

What is the cure? In many cases, where a back aches simply because it has not been exercised and has therefore lost muscle tone, exercise is the obvious answer. For more severe cases, muscle-building exercises conscientiously carried out can restore the back to the point that it will not give pain unless it is again injured or abused.

But because many people resist the idea of exercise, back sufferers have been shopping for years for a magical cure, from the traditional mustard plaster to electric heating pads, diathermy, ultrasound, massage, manipulation by osteopaths or chiropractors, injections of anesthetics or papaya extracts, water beds, mud beds, acupuncture, yoga, and hypnotism. Some of these techniques are legitimate, others fraudulent.

According to a joint study by Columbia University and New York University of 5,000 consecutive patients with low-back complaints, 81 per cent had no skeletal disorders—nothing wrong with either bones or discs. Instead, their pains were all traceable to muscles, ligaments, or tendons, and were the outcome of strains, sprains, poor posture, or lack of exercise.

If a backache victim has no skeletal disorder, surgery will do nothing for him. And even among those people who have skeletal disorders, up to 90 per cent still do not need surgery. In other words, physicians are almost unanimous as to the value of "conservative management" and exercise for the backache victim.

After the patient has left the hospital, the burden is his to keep himself in shape so that his back doesn't bother him again. Doctors agree that at least thirty minutes of exercise per day is mandatory, all at once or in two sessions. There is controversy, however, about which specific exercises are the most helpful. Generally, each specialist in orthopedics or physical medicine has developed his own set of exercises.

Some 140 muscles are involved in supporting the back and controlling its movement, and far from all of them are in the back area. Of the four most important groups supporting the back, one set is out in front—the abdominal muscles. People who walk around with sagging stomachs are also dragging down their spines; the simple act of tightening these muscles frequently will strengthen the back in the long run.

Eminent New York physician Dr. Howard A. Rusk, head of the Institute of Rehabilitation Medicine, notes that many back-strengthening exercises can be carried out inconspicuously while standing in a line or sitting on a train: for example, the "pelvic thrust" or "tucking your tail under" or tightening your abdominal muscles. Such simple maneuvers, combined with a daily half hour of exercise, should put an end to all back problems. But consistency is essential.

Stand up straight

Unnecessary fatigue often troubles people who have "occupational postures"—barbers, truck drivers, musicians, cleaning women. These people must make an effort to compensate for their habits by purposely using different muscles. Postural problems are also evident among people who have simply never learned to hold their bodies properly.

Since our bodies are flexible, we can easily stand on one leg, flop into a chair, sit on one foot, or curl up on a couch without doing any damage. Nevertheless, if one or more of these positions becomes habitual, it is easy to develop some postures that feel comfortable even though they include round shoulders, sway-back, a high hip, or a forward head.

Sitting and standing are forms of exercise, just as swimming or bowling are, and they are just as important as the more obvious forms of exercise. The changes a person can make in his appearance depend on learning new habits in using the body as well as on exercise in areas needing special attention.

Here are the American Medical Association's recommendations for developing better posture:

When Standing:
- Feet slightly apart, weight balanced on both feet, toes straight ahead;
- Knees straight, relaxed;
- Hips tucked, abdomen flat;
- Chest slightly up and forward;
- Neck and head balanced over the body, chin in; stretch up at the back of the neck and head.

When Walking:
- Toes straight ahead;
- Feet parallel and close together as you step;
- Push forward with the back foot;
- Control the length of the step for an even, rhythmic stride;
- Place the heel first in stepping, followed by the outside portion of the sole and by the forefoot;
- Swing arms easily.

When Sitting:
- Feet flat on floor;
- Thighs supported by chair as far as the curve of the knee;
- Back supported by chair back, body straight from hips to neck.

When Working:
- Stand erect, balanced and relaxed;
- Correct working heights to prevent slumping or excessive reaching;
- When lifting, stand close to the object; draw it close to your center of gravity; lift with the strong muscles of legs and shoulders; shift body balance at base to accommodate added weight.

Map out an exercise program

The best kind of exercise is based on regular activity that uses many parts of the body, that is rigorous enough to tax muscle power, and that can be done long enough and strenuously enough to produce a sense of healthful fatigue.

These requirements can be fulfilled in different ways, according to a person's age and physical condition. Check with your doctor if you have not been exercising regularly for a long time or if you have had any serious health problems. Use common sense: Don't start playing touch football after twenty years of ping-pong.

The AMA recommends that an exercise program be approached from three directions:

Plan a regular schedule. The serious exerciser should set aside at least half an hour per day at least five days per week, during which time wild horses cannot tear him away from his athletic activities. He should come to consider this part of his life as essential as eating or sleeping.

Many people have become discouraged with their failure to lose weight after conscientiously following an exercise program. There are two considerations to this problem: first, adjustments in metabolism take place slowly, and it may be a while before the difference is noticeable on the scale. Second, muscle tissue weighs more than flabby tissue; it also takes up less space. Thus it is possible to weigh more and yet look better.

Look for supplementary recreation. In addition to carrying out a regular program of exercise, look for the unscheduled event which will also give you a chance to use your body. Go on a fishing trip with the next-door neighbor, go dancing at the local club, take the children to the zoo.

Step up your daily activities. Bend, stoop, stretch, squat, reach, move, lift, carry. Walk to the grocery store; park several blocks from work; walk up stairs instead of using the elevator; stand up to put on and remove stockings and shoes. Look for opportunities to use your body, and avoid time-saving devices that rob you of the chance to burn off a few calories. Instead of considering an errand downstairs or a trip to the other side of the building as an annoyance, think of it as an added boost to fitness.

Although these little efforts do not cost very much energy in themselves, they can add up to an appreciable calorie drain by the end of the day. Also, they can contribute significantly to improved muscle tone, flexibility, and balance.

The no-sweat exercises

In recent years much publicity has been given to isometric exercises, whose promoters have made a number of exaggerated claims—for example, that with only five minutes of exercise per day you can increase your strength, broaden your shoulders, reduce your waistline, and increase your lung capacity. Isometrics, so the advertising goes, are ideal for people who have neither the time, the space, nor the interest for a regular exercise program.

Unfortunately, the value of isometrics as a fitness aid has been vastly overrated, and many of the gadgets sold commercially for "muscle-building" are virtually useless.

In order to obtain the strength-building benefits of isometric exercise, it is necessary to reach close to a maximum contraction of the muscle. The isometric exercises touted in popular magazines come nowhere near this point.

Isometrics are not recommended as the basis of a fitness program for another reason: It would take a great deal of time to do a proper job. These exercises are very specific, and one would have to work each part of the body separately in order to get a complete workout.

Despite its limitations, however, isometric exercise does serve a function. It is especially helpful for people who are immobilized and who cannot exercise normally. Isometrics are also valuable as spot reducers; for example, they are often recommended for a woman who has just had a child and whose stomach muscles are flabby.

Can yoga keep you in shape?

For the past hundred years, interest in the practice of yoga has waxed and waned in this country. The current burst of enthusiasm can be traced largely to Western interest in Oriental philosophy and in the martial arts such as karate and judo. Generally, much less attention is paid to the philosophical aspects of yoga than to its physical practices.

Yoga devotees speak highly of its tension-reducing effects and the improvements in body flexibility which accompany regular practice. One authoritative source, Dr. Allan J. Ryan, points out, however, "The available evidence relating to the theory and practice of yoga does not indicate that it makes any positive contribution to the development of physical fitness as we understand it, with the possible exception of the improvement in flexibility." Dr. Ryan, an orthopedic surgeon, is chief athletic physician at the University of Wisconsin.

A beginner is usually able to master the postural and breathing techniques within six to twelve weeks, while proper performance of the more difficult postures may take as long as three years.

"The postural activities are not supposed to be exercises in the ordinary sense, since their purpose is to stretch the body and relax tension, not to build muscle size or strength," Dr. Ryan points out. "The values of calisthenics and sports in this regard are indeed derided by serious practitioners of yoga."

Obviously, specific muscles may become stronger as a result of maintaining certain positions for extended periods; however, these muscle groups may not influence overall strength as it is normally measured.

Evidence relating to change in cardiac function as the result of yoga practice is meager and partially contradictory, he comments. "There is no reason to believe from a conceptual analysis of yoga practices that the ability of the heart to increase the efficiency of the circulation or to recover from strenuous exercise is improved."

In fact, he adds, many yoga practitioners feel that each person's heart is allotted only a certain number of beats for a lifetime and that speeding of the heart by vigorous exercise may only hasten that person's death.

Obviously, then, yoga cannot be counted on for the kind of physical conditioning that would make a University of Wisconsin football player. On the other hand, many people find it an excellent form of relaxation and an antidote to fatigue. Others consider it boring and would much rather be out smashing a badminton bird.

BIBLIOGRAPHY

"The ABC's of Perfect Posture," American Medical Association pamphlet. Chicago, 1967.

Cant, Gilbert. "Our Aching Backs!" *New York Times Magazine,* Feb. 3, 1974.

"Exercise and Weight Control," American Medical Association pamphlet. Chicago.

Gendel, Evalyn S., M.D. "Women: Fitness and Fatigue," *West Virginia Medical Journal,* May 1973.

Guild, Warren R., M.D. "Don't Laugh—Physical Fitness Can Be Fun," *MD's Wife,* July 1970.

Higdon, Hal. "Let's Tell the Truth About Isometrics," *Today's Health,* June 1965.

Lentz, John J. "To Exercise or Not to Exercise?" *Today's Health,* Mar. 1963.

"Physical Fitness," American Medical Association pamphlet. Chicago, 1969.

Ryan, Allan J., M.D. "Yoga and Fitness," *Journal of Health, Physical Education, Recreation,* Feb. 1971.

White, Paul Dudley, M.D. "Physical Exercise," Massachusetts Heart Association, Inc., pamphlet, Jan. 1969.

6 YOU ARE WHAT YOU EAT

Back in high school, many of us sat through nutrition classes led by a little lady who pulled her hair back into a hairnet and dressed neat as a pin. Using a wooden pointer, she introduced us to "the basic seven," working her way around a chart cut into seven wedges, each one illustrating the foods in that category.

In those days we ate enough food anyway, so that we probably were getting most of our nutrient requirements, in addition to the caloric overflow provided by after-school ice cream sodas and midnight raids on the refrigerator. But as time goes on, the urgings of the nutritionists fall upon indifferent ears; after all, we figure that as adults we should know what is good for us without being told.

So diet habits become slipshod; calories once expended on milk are now consumed in scotch, an apple after lunch is replaced by coffee loaded with cream and sugar. Many people spend most of their lives agonizing through one reducing diet after another, usually one of the high-protein, low-carbohydrate diets which have won the devotion of millions. These diet fanatics are conditioned to think of certain perfectly nutritious foods as off limits. Bananas and oranges are for special occasions; breads and cereals, forever untouchable.

All of which is to say: No matter how much you know about proper eating, chances are you aren't applying your knowledge. And fatigue is a frequent by-product of poor eating habits.

Our lamentable eating patterns

As anyone can testify who has gone a long time without a decent meal, being very hungry makes a person very tired, and also puts him in a menacing, irritable frame of mind. The body, deprived of blood sugar, is temporarily "out of gas." Although plenty of fuel is stored in body fat, this reserve cannot be drawn upon easily.

At this point it is the instinct of many people to rush to the nearest vending machine, shove in a dime and swallow a Hershey bar or a Peter Paul Almond Joy. This raises the blood sugar level and provides quick energy, but a letdown period tends to follow close on the heels of the candy high.

A more intelligent means of subduing hunger pangs is to sit down and eat a substantial snack—something with food value such as a cup of soup, a hamburger, or a piece of fruit. First, real food provides more long-term energy than "junk food"; second, the brief pause in itself refreshes much more than the handful of potato chips eaten while running for the bus or standing over the ironing board.

The "three square meals a day" philosophy has been drummed into the American child; his parents are often guilty of a double standard. Three square meals is essential for the kids, but one is enough for their elders. The mother, if she is at home, tends to sample what she is preparing for the children, or eat what they leave. The thought of whipping up a gourmet lunch to eat alone is not enticing, so she heats up a cup of bouillon and takes the cottage cheese from the refrigerator. The husband, or the woman who works, has neither the time, interest, nor the appetite to sit around eating oatmeal in the morning while the kids pull each other's hair. By the time he or she gets into the office, the day has sufficiently fallen into place that he can relax with a cup of coffee and a prune Danish.

The prune Danish has little staying power, but the office person is leery of eating a big lunch. After all, there is the prospect of cocktails at 5:30 and there's that big dinner party at the next-door neighbors'.

So calories are hoarded for a grand finale at the end of the day, when they are least needed. The end result: The blood is overloaded with fat at a time when no effort will be exerted to burn it off. It stays with the consumer, who is often too tired to work off dinner even if he had time. After a very large meal, too much of the blood supply is busy trying to digest and absorb the food. Blood is diverted from the brain, and one becomes sleepy and sluggish.

Both obese people and excessively thin people become tired more quickly than the rest of the population. The fat person needs extra energy to move his bulky frame around, and the thin person may not have enough reserve fuel on his body to take him over long periods without food and rest. The obvious answer is to lose or gain weight, whichever is necessary. Granted, this is easier said than done.

What does the average adult need to stay healthy, slim, and free of fatigue? Following is a summary of the Basic Four food groups and the daily adult requirements for each:

The Milk Group
• Two or more servings per day.
• Includes milk in all forms, cheese, ice cream, yoghurt.
• Milk is a main source of calcium, and also provides protein, riboflavin, vitamin A and other nutrients.

The Meat Group
• Two or more servings per day.
• Includes beef, veal, lamb, pork, variety meats such as liver, heart, kidney; poultry, eggs, fish, shellfish, dried beans or peas, soybeans, lentils, nuts.
• These foods are valued chiefly for their protein content, but they also provide iron, thiamine, riboflavin, and niacin.

The Vegetable/Fruit Group
• One serving from the following: deep-green or deep-yellow vegetables, such as broccoli, carrots, sweet potatoes.
• One serving from the following: citrus fruits, tomatoes, and other fruits rich in vitamin C such as berries; vegetables such as cauliflower, asparagus, green peppers.

• One serving of the following: potatoes, pineapples, apples, bananas, beets, lima beans, corn.

• One other serving from the first or second groups above.

• This group is the primary source of vitamins and minerals in the diet.

The Bread/Cereal Group

• Three to four servings per day.

• Includes bread, cereal, pastas, rice, corn meal, grits, crackers, muffins, biscuits, pancakes, waffles, cookies, cakes.

• If you are dieting, eliminate the caloric members of this group, but not all. These foods provide iron, vitamins, carbohydrates and protein.

In addition, you will be expected to use some butter or fortified margarine on your food. Mayonnaise, salad dressings, and cooking oils also provide necessary fats in the diet.

Alcohol

Where do hard liquor, wine, and beer fit into the nutritional picture?

Distilled liquors such as gin, whiskey, vodka, and brandy are heavy with calories, and they also stimulate the appetite. A cocktail or two before dinner will not harm most people, but too much alcohol dulls the taste of food and encourages a craving for fatty foods.

"Experienced cocktail party habitués learn that their staying power is improved by eating fatty foods which slow the absorption of alcohol, but we doubt that this is the best way of preserving both sobriety and health," Dr. Ancel Keys counsels in *Eat Well and Stay Well.*

"At the cocktail party, take highballs with much soda instead of short drinks, or, even better, take white wine and soda as a good way of controlling the alcohol intake."

Years ago it was discovered that the arteries of chronic alcoholics are often surprisingly free of atherosclerosis. Prosperous, well-fed alcoholics are not, however, specially protected from heart disease. Many chronic drunkards are seriously undernourished, and thus are not eating the foods that lead to deposits of fat and cholesterol in the arterial walls. Also, their livers cannot make very much cholesterol or blood fat.

The medical eye perceives few virtues in hard liquor, although it is unlikely that it will disappear from the American scene for that reason. Wine is another story, however. More and more Americans are discovering that wine with dinner complements the best cooking, enlivens even dull food, and generally contributes to an atmosphere of gracious living. Also, it easily replaces fat in its moistening effects, and excellent low-fat sauces can be made with wine.

"All honest dry wines have a place at the civilized table," Dr. Keys maintains. "Sweet wines are something else; they have their uses, particularly with desserts on special occasions, but they should not be used before or during the main part of a meal if you hope to savor either food or wine flavors."

If you are serving a good wine with dinner, try to encourage your guests to take a glass of vermouth with lemon peel or some dry sherry rather than a heavy cocktail beforehand. This will keep tastes sharp and heads sober.

Beer lacks the subtleties, gastronomic credentials, and snob appeal of wine, but it has a lot of supporters. "Beer has a special affinity for raw oysters, but otherwise it goes best with plain, hearty, fatty foods that have little place in a cuisine designed to let you eat well and stay well," Dr. Keys says. "But you may disagree, and we have no objection to beer in your diet provided you count your calories."

Beer contains a wide range of nutrients, although in small concentrations. It also has a lot of carbohydrates. Alcohol content is not high: The average person needs to drink quite a lot, and very quickly, to get drunk.

The AHA lifetime diet

The American Heart Association is the moving force in a campaign to change the American diet by reducing cholesterol and raising polyunsaturated fats in our diet, thus lowering the rates of obesity, high blood pressure, and heart disease. Recently the AHA published a large, glossy cookbook which includes AHA-approved recipes along with charts and data on food composition.

Recommendations are based on the 1957 Prudent Diet, which was the outcome of efforts of the Anti-Coronary Club of the New York City Health Department. The Prudent Diet has been the backbone of the AHA philosophy since that time.

The organization is concerned about diet because about one million Americans are struck by coronary heart disease each year, of whom almost two thirds die immediately. Of the several factors which contribute to heart disease—age, stress, smoking habits, sex, heredity, and diet—the last is the easiest to modify; hence the all-out effort at prevention.

Although heart attacks used to strike middle-aged men more than anyone else, in recent years the number of younger male victims has been on the rise, and more women have been struck as well. In fact, autopsies of soldiers in both Vietnam and Korea showed that twenty-year-old men had arteries as blocked as those of men more than twice their age. Obviously, then, the destructive process begins very early, and good eating habits should begin in earliest childhood.

The AHA makes a number of recommendations which can be applied across the board to the typical American family:

• Cut 25 per cent off daily calorie intake by eliminating junk foods of little nutritional value—popcorn, candy, potato chips, etc. Also, go easy on desserts, pastries, fatty meats, beer, sweet wines, hard liquors, and soft drinks with sugar added.

• Reduce cholesterol intake: no more than four egg yolks a week for adults and seven for children, including those used in cooking; limit use of shellfish, organ meats, and fatty "variety meats" such as bacon, sausage, corned beef, pastrami, salami, sausages.

• The main course at lunch or dinner should include: fish five times a week, shellfish not more than twice, poultry several times (but don't fry it and don't eat the skin). Meat should be restricted to four servings per week for a total of sixteen ounces or less. Veal is an excellent choice, as it has so little fat. If you use beef, lamb, pork, or ham, cut off all visible fat.

• Instead of butter and other cooking fats that are solid or completely hydrogenated, use liquid vegetable oils and margarines that are rich in polyunsaturated fats. Avoid the use of fats in cooking and instead use cooking methods that help to remove fat: bake, boil, broil, roast, stew. Don't eat gravy or rich sauces.

• Milk-drinking adults should limit themselves to a pint of skimmed or low-fat milk per day. Children may drink a pint of whole milk, but beyond that should join parents in the low-fat variety.

• Total of such high-fat cheeses as cheddar, American, Swiss, and Camembert should not exceed four ounces per week. Cottage, pot, and farmer cheese are low in fat and high in protein, thus usage is strongly encouraged. Sweet cream, sour cream, cream cheese, and ice cream are also on the list of undesirables.

• Whole-grain or enriched bread or cereal may be used with every meal, and nuts, seeds, and beans can be served frequently. Dark-green, leafy, and deep-yellow vegetables should appear on the menu at least four times a week. Everybody should have high-vitamin C fruit or juice every day (orange, tomato, grapefruit, cantaloupe).

In recent years many Americans have heeded the AHA's advice and switched to polyunsaturated fats for most cooking. Yet the total fat consumed per capita continues to fly high—it is estimated that each one of us consumes fifty-three pounds per year of "straight" fats—butter, lard, margarine, shortening, salad oils.

Reaching the AHA's goal of deriving fewer than 35 per cent of total calories from fat sources would necessitate drastic reductions in the amount of foods containing "invisible" fats—meat, eggs, dairy products.

Americans also consume about a hundred pounds of refined sugar per person per year, most of it coming from manufactured foods and 23 per cent from beverages. Nutritionists generally agree that this is too much, and that we should either lose our taste for sweets or use noncaloric artificial sweeteners. With cyclamates outlawed and saccharin threatened, however, few alternatives are available.

The "ideal" breakfast

John, a corporate lawyer, is clutching the sports page of the morning paper in one hand and spooning oatmeal into his mouth with the other. A half-eaten grapefruit rests on a plate to the side.

Betty, his pregnant wife, has already finished her grapefruit and is delving enthusiastically into two scrambled eggs with cheese and an English muffin. She reaches for a jar of her aunt's homemade peach preserves.

Roberta, John's seventeen-year-old daughter by a previous marriage, is sipping black coffee and studying a shorthand manual. She is taking a summer course at the local high school in preparation for university.

Who is eating the "proper" breakfast? Everybody, according to Dr. Jean Mayer, the widely published professor of nutrition at Harvard University and a leading food expert. Although our ears have been filled with the virtues of eating a big breakfast to start the day with lots of energy, many healthy and energetic people eat almost nothing in the morning, notes Dr. Mayer, who was chairman of the 1969 First White House Conference on Food, Nutrition and Health.

"I realize this may sound almost sacrilegious—after all, Theodore Roosevelt set the national example when he declared that 'Good men eat breakfast,'" Dr. Mayer comments. "So often people ask me: 'Just what is a good breakfast?' Sadly, there's no simple answer: it all depends upon your activity and your physical health, including blood cholesterol and weight."

The classic American morning fare—orange juice, cereal, eggs, bacon, toast, and milk—is fine if you are a nursing mother or a very active growing child. But for most people, this kind of eating should be reserved for the occasional Sunday morning at a small country inn.

Everybody needs vitamin C, which the body cannot store; thus a daily glass of fruit juice or a piece of grapefruit is good advice. If you don't get your vitamin C in the morning, be sure to eat some fruit later in the day, he suggests.

Cereal is also a good idea, particularly for people on low-fat low-cholesterol diets. John adores hot oatmeal or cream of wheat with a touch of brown sugar and a splash of whole milk. His doctor is trying to convert him to skim milk to eliminate the unnecessary fats in whole milk, but so far he hasn't been able to make the switch, nor is he too concerned, as his total diet is fairly low in fats.

As a child, Roberta was addicted to the cold processed cereals heavily coated with sugar and more interesting for the games and puzzles on the back of the box than for the contents. She has since shunned these uninteresting and unnutritious sources of excess calories.

What about eggs? They are fine for Betty, who is thirty-two years old and well below the age where cholesterol becomes a problem for a woman. They are a good source of iron, too, of which pregnant women need as much as they can get.

John has been leery of eggs for several years now, ever since he learned that his blood cholesterol level was 250, considerably higher than the 220 which many physicians consider the safe level. Research indicates that men with cholesterol levels as high as 300 stand a much better chance of having a heart attack, although a low cholesterol level is no guarantee that you won't have one. Cholesterol in food will raise blood cholesterol levels; however, a person with high blood cholesterol who eliminates eggs from his diet will not necessarily drop to the safe point.

"The best course for egg lovers would seem to be to know your cholesterol level," Dr. Mayer suggests. "If it is under 200, in spite of your eating two eggs a day, you obviously are able to handle them. If not, adopt a more prudent diet or try a cholesterol-free egg substitute."

Bacon is fine as an occasional treat, but it is high in calories and fat and limited in protein.

Need for variety

While many people sing the praises of the first meal of the day, others are completely unenthusiastic, partly because the breakfast menu in most homes and restaurants is so predictable—eggs-and-bacon or pancakes-and-syrup. Dr. Mayer suggests that a little more imagination on the part of the meal planner might result in more enthusiasm for the meal.

For example, why not serve the leftovers from last night's dinner? Or perhaps a tray of cheeses, interesting breads, and cold meats? Children particularly are not hung up on eating certain foods at certain hours of the day, and they may exhibit an encouraging change of appetite if offered a tuna fish sandwich in place of a soft-boiled egg and toast.

Some studies have suggested that adults who eat a good breakfast work more productively and for a longer period than those who omit or skimp on the meal. Also, teachers have reported that well-breakfasted children have a better overall attitude, are more attentive and score better grades than those who eat nothing.

Still, the matter remains an individual one. Roberta wants nothing more than black coffee at 8 A.M., but at ten o'clock she is ready for orange juice and a bran muffin. Children present a different problem. Although in general they are much better off with a substantial meal before leaving home, some children are not hungry first thing in the morning and simply will not eat breakfast if rushed.

"This is particularly true of small children—say, kindergarten through the second or third grade," Dr. Mayer points out. "They either have to get up very early (often a traumatic experience for the whole family) or they have to be fed after they arrive at school (some schools now serve breakfast before the first class, although the quality of the breakfast is not always ideal)."

Dr. Mayer recommends that if you cannot get your child to eat a good breakfast, then give him an extra sandwich to eat in school at the midmorning milk or juice break. Otherwise he will not have energy to get him through to lunch.

The same does not hold true for adults, however. Various studies notwithstanding, how well adults function with or without a morning meal seems to depend largely on what they are used to. People who are accustomed to a substantial meal in the morning feel very empty by midmorning if unfed. But in some European countries, the thought of a large breakfast is almost revolting to people used to a cup of coffee with cream and a sweet roll with butter.

At the other extreme, in many parts of Africa people eat only one meal a day—in the evenings. Although they grab an occasional snack in the daylight hours, the serious eating is reserved for a long, elaborate evening feast. On the other hand, the inhabitants of the Pacific islands have few organized meals at any time.

"Hence, as we look at the world at large, we see that our three meals a day is the exception rather than the rule and that the first meal of the day, in particular, is extremely variable," Dr. Mayer observes.

The nutrition question aside, a good breakfast can serve as a point of contact for families who often spend a minimum of time together. In a household where everybody is on a different schedule and where a family dinner is often sacrificed to the demands of professional and civic obligations, breakfast together can serve as a treasured time for communication.

"Even if you are one of those adults who can function well with a light breakfast, you'll find the day gets off to a more satisfactory start if you arrange to share a few early-morning moments with your family," Dr. Mayer declares.

How crash diets drain your energy

Next time you're sitting on the bus or waiting in line at the movies, take a good look around and see if you don't agree with the findings of a recent U. S. Public Health survey: At least one American adult in every four is more than 20 per cent overweight.

Not everybody finds billowing rolls of flesh distasteful; some people like the full-blown look. But in twentieth-century America fat is definitely not chic, and although few women can approximate the gaunt look of a fashion model, that look is the modern image of beauty.

Whether fat is ugly is a matter of taste; however, it can certainly be both physically and psychologically uncomfortable. Obese youngsters, for example, often see themselves as a member of a minority group and the object of subtle discrimination.

Although a few pounds too many are not physically harmful, people who are grossly overweight are recognized medical risks. They have higher rates of liver disease, diabetes, hypertension, appendicitis, gall bladder disease, and accidental death.

In case that's not enough bad news, an American Cancer Society study of 800,000 people indicates that obese people have one and a half to three and a half times as many fatal heart attacks and strokes as normal people.

Dr. Ancel Keys, who has been a prominent researcher in heart disease for many years, stresses that no one has proved that being fat in itself can lead to heart disease. "Obesity is common in Italy, but coronary heart disease is relatively rare; in England, coronary heart disease is almost as prevalent as in the United States, but obesity is much less frequent than here or in Italy. We have no doubt, however, that obesity is a hazard to health in other directions . . . if you are fat, you should reduce."

Certainly the litany is a familiar one: Eat sensibly and you will look better, feel better, and live longer. What does all of this have to do with fatigue? First, fat people tire easily, because they have all that weight to drag around. Grotesquely obese people will be even more exhausted because their bodies operate inefficiently; fat gets in the way of normal motions such as the swinging of an arm.

Another link between weight and fatigue is that fat or nearly fat people are often on diets—poorly conceived, nutritionally unsound regimens which leave the dieter mentally and physically run down. This fatigue breeds indifference or self-pity, which propels the dieter back to the kitchen.

Since the ranks of Americans who are either obese or on a bad diet are legion, a lot of people should probably be reading this chapter.

Obesity research

Experts are offering a variety of theories about how we as a nation have arrived at a state of overnourishment (although it should be noted that malnutrition arising from poverty is far from a rare phenomenon in this country). Many pediatricians maintain that our babies are too well fed; they get used to eating a lot from the beginning, and the habit remains ingrained.

The old rule of thumb held that a baby should double his birth weight by six months and triple it by one year, but infants fed rich liquid formulas and solid foods early in life regularly surpass this limit.

Some researchers say that the person who habitually consumes more calories than he burns has suffered a derangement of the hypothalamus, which regulates the sensations of hunger and fullness. The evidence, so far almost wholly provided by animal studies, remains inconclusive.

Others have suggested that fat people eat too much because they have a low blood sugar condition called hypoglycemia. This theory is particularly popular among authors of diet books, but scientists who study carbohydrate metabolism do not agree. Some feel that when an obese person undergoes the symptoms of hypoglycemia—rapid heartbeat, perspiration, and shakiness—he is more likely to be suffering from anxiety, which is also triggered by excess amounts of epinephrine (adrenalin) in the bloodstream.

Several studies indicate that fat people have defective or nonexistent sensations of hunger, that they do not receive the normal signs—such as a growling stomach—that say it's time to eat, and that they, consequently, do not know when it's time to stop.

Habitual overeaters are also extremely responsive to external cues. For example, if it is 12 noon and they are used to eating lunch at that time, they will eat. Thin people will eat then only if they are hungry. Obese people glut themselves; their opposites eat only what satisfies them. The fatties are also turned on by the sight of food. If they pass by a bakery, they cannot resist the enchantments displayed in the window. Their thin friends can stroll nonchalantly by.

"Not only do the obese eat more than lean individuals, they seem to be less active," notes Dr. Richard F. Spark, assistant clinical professor of medicine at Harvard Medical School. "For example, when pedometers are attached to lean and obese housewives, the lean housewives will walk twice as far, although they are presumably engaged in the same types of activity."

How much to lose?

One way to judge whether you should be thinking about dropping a few pounds is to try the "pinch test." Grasp the flesh just above your waist between the thumb and the tip of the forefinger. If the accumulation measures more than an inch or so in thickness, take a good look in the mirror. Possibly you need to lose a few pounds, although possibly your body build is such that you have extra flesh at the waist while the rest looks fine. In that case, exercise is the answer. (Certainly, exercise is a necessity for all dieters, if they don't want their fat to sag unattractively as they lose weight.)

There is really no one ideal weight for a particular height, only a range. Much depends on how your weight looks on you. Some people can get away with an extra fifteen pounds; others look fleshy at only a few pounds to the wrong side.

Calories, despite their bad reputation, are nothing more than units of heat energy. The average person who leads a moderately active life needs 15 calories per pound of body weight to maintain his desired weight. In other words, a woman who looks good and is happy at 150 pounds should run a calorie total of no more than 2,250 calories per day ($150 \times 15 = 2,250$).

The dieter must cut a considerable chunk out of his calorie budget, although without necessarily reducing the amount of food consumed. Each pound of stored body fat contains some 3,500 calories. This means that in order to lose two pounds per week, you will have to cut back by 1,000 calories per day from the norm. In other words, our 150-pound lady would have to go on a diet of 1,250 calories per day in order to lose her two pounds.

Doctors recommend that people aim at losing no more than this amount; otherwise, the pounds have a tendency to sneak back quickly, and the dieter may find himself tired, ill-humored, and more susceptible to illness.

If all the books and articles written about dieting were stacked on top of each other, the pile would probably reach to the moon. It is not the purpose of this book to give detailed instructions on how to lose weight, but because the dieter is such easy prey to fatigue and discouragement, a few words about mental attitude are in order.

Overweight is a frustrating problem for everyone—for the victims as well as the doctors trying to help them. Most "dramatic weight loss" stories have an unhappy ending. The person who did the unbelievable and lost a hundred pounds is right back at the same "fat farm" the following year, fat as ever. Moderately overweight people also tend to bounce back and forth; many never reach a point of equilibrium, but are either on a diet or on a binge.

For the truly obese this ping-pong game is not only discouraging, it is dangerous. The body organs get attuned to functioning for a person at a certain weight; the sudden and frequent jolts provided by periods of loss and gain put great stress on these organs.

Yet the ping-pong game is not inevitable. We are cursed with an inheritance of fat-making food habits, but it is never too late to unlearn if the rewards are sufficient. Psychologically, the serious dieter must prepare to give up some old habits forever. This means he shouldn't embark on a reducing program unless he is dead serious —halfhearted efforts leave damaged egos when the efforts fail.

For many people, reducing groups such as Weight Watchers provide invaluable support and direction, while others prefer reducing under the watchful eye of their doctor. The majority of dieters go it alone. However you start, don't forget that it is possible to change. Somehow, everybody can lose weight.

The great vitamin debate

According to a recent survey by the U. S. Food and Drug Administration, guardian of national sanity in drug usage, more than sixty million Americans believe that vitamin supplements are necessary to maintain normal health. Some twenty million are convinced that vitamin deficiency is the cause of most illness in this country.

Scientists have been arguing the merits of vitamins for years—how much of these mysterious substances are needed by the normal adult and whether massive doses are harmful, helpful, or merely ineffective. Yet despite a remarkable lack of conclusive evidence, at least one person in 75 per cent of U.S. households has taken vitamins, and 80 per cent of these are regular users.

The fact that vitamins are so important, that they function in various ways, and that they are easily available in pill form has opened wide the doors to people looking for miracle drugs, and for people willing to sell them. Although as recently as thirty years ago the belief was widespread that vitamins were harmless and could be taken in huge amounts, that naïve theory has been called sharply into question.

For nearly ten years the Food and Drug Administration listened to arguments on both sides of the vitamin controversy. Their efforts were spurred largely by the realization that Americans were spending more than $300 million annually for vitamin and mineral products whose effects were not clearly defined.

The debate ended in the publication in August, 1973, of a massive series of regulations on the labeling, sale, and promotion of vitamins and minerals. As expected, the new regulations raised cries of protest from vitamin addicts, and the FDA was dragged immediately into litigation on various issues stemming from the new rules.

In response to its critics, the FDA insisted that no vitamins would be taken off the market completely, and that none would become exclusively prescription drugs.

In only two cases—vitamins A and D—were vitamins redefined as prescription items, and these restrictions apply only to high-strength pills that give the user more than the recommended daily allowance: for vitamin D, 400 international units and for vitamin

A, 1,500–8,000 units (infants and nursing mothers representing the two extremes). Pills containing more than 10,000 international units of vitamin A or 400 units of vitamin D can only be obtained with a prescription. There is nothing to stop a devotee from stuffing himself on smaller amounts. Regulations for other drugs are less strict.

Vitamin E

This is the vitamin which has received the most publicity and about which the most exaggerated claims have been made. As Dr. Keys puts it, "Vitamin E has been the subject of more nonsensical claims than most vitamins—which is saying a lot . . . Alas! dosing with vitamin E and wheat-germ oil seems to be only one more futile gesture in the age-old search for fertility and virility."

Vitamin E, discovered sixty years ago, has not been proved necessary for man. "If you are concerned about getting enough vitamin E, don't bother with taking pills, just use a lot of corn oil and cottonseed oil," Dr. Keys advises.

Millions of Americans swallow large doses of this vitamin every day or smear it on their skin in the hopes that it will cure diseases from acne to heart conditions. An estimated eight hundred tons go into products for human use in this country each year.

Although skeptics can sneer at the gullibility of a nation seduced by a pharmaceutical industry, even doses of fifty times the recommended daily allowances of vitamin E have so far produced no side effects. Thus many physicians are unwilling to deprive patients who are "hooked" on them, on the theory that "it can't hurt."

"If you take away their vitamin E, some patients get very depressed and uncomfortable—it's their security blanket, so I let them have it," Dr. M. K. Horwitt, a pioneer in human vitamin E research, admits.

Dr. Horwitt, who is professor of biochemistry at St. Louis University School of Medicine, feels that vitamin E is not harmful as long as the patient can afford it and as long as he is not using it in place of a standard drug needed to treat illness.

Recently the prestigious National Academy of Sciences condemned the national obsession with vitamins, claiming that many assertions of their value were based on preliminary animal research.

According to NAS's Committee on Nutritional Misinformation, there is no scientific evidence of value that vitamin E can promote physical endurance, enhance sexual potency, prevent heart attacks, protect against air pollution, slow the aging process, or perform any other miraculous feats.

Vitamin E, which has been labeled the "vitamin in search of a disease," has also been cited as a cure for cancer, muscular dystrophy, ulcers, sterility, burns, skin disorders, and lung disease.

In what fertile soil do such exaggerated claims take root? Certainly, people are too eager to jump to conclusions from scanty evidence. When vitamin E deficiency is induced in animals, definite pathological changes can result, but it is difficult as well as unethical to set up similar experiments in human beings; thus the limited amount of testing has been inconclusive.

Investigators have also found that white male rats deprived of food containing vitamin E will become sterile. Yet this by no means indicates that the same would happen to man, nor that excessive doses of the drug will cure sterility, as some have wistfully hoped.

And although severe vitamin E deficiency causes muscle wasting in most animals studied, levels of this substance are normal in persons with muscular dystrophy. Pumping them up with vitamin E does nothing for their disease.

According to the NAS committee, supplementary vitamin E has proved useful in only two situations: for premature babies who were not getting enough of the vitamin before birth, and for people with malabsorption syndromes such as cystic fibrosis and blockage of the bile duct in which fats are poorly absorbed. The rest of us might as well throw out the bottle.

Because of the sensational aspects of the vitamin E debate, aired widely in the press, many researchers have tried to stay clear of it. This presents a stumbling block to serious investigation. Another problem hindering more conclusive findings: It is difficult to find a person whose diet is truly deficient in vitamin E.

Even when salad oils and whole-grain foods are eliminated, it takes a long time for vitamin E levels to drop. In fact, after many months on a vitamin E-deficient diet, most people show only a small reduction in the lifetimes of their red blood cells.

Vitamin C

The name Linus Pauling has been added to the list of household words; few educated Americans are unfamiliar with the dictates of the Nobel prize-winning chemist and staunch peace advocate who in 1970 published *Vitamin C and the Common Cold.* According to Dr. Pauling, massive doses of ascorbic acid (vitamin C) will prevent colds and let you live longer. Naturally, sales of his book scored stupendous highs, and throngs of admirers formed to his rear.

Many of Dr. Pauling's critics argue that his megavitamin theory won't work because people will simply excrete the excess. Others fear that the excessive quantities may lead to complications such as the formation of stones in the urinary tract.

Dr. Pauling replies that excretion is not a problem. Heavy doses of a water-soluble vitamin such as C, taken regularly, set up a steady state in the body, which adapts to the influx. As for side effects, he quotes studies indicating that up to 100 grams of the nutrient cause no such effects.

If the vitamin capsules are dropped into an empty stomach, mild gastric upset may result, he cautions. Nevertheless, many of the cold cures on the market produce a similar reaction.

Scientists argue that Dr. Pauling made only nineteen studies of the effect of vitamin C on colds, most of which concluded that the vitamin had negligible positive results. Pauling does not agree with this interpretation. Subjects showed fewer colds in the studies, he says, even though they were taking less than the recommended dose.

His detractors also claim that the two large studies on which he lays the burden of proof were not conducted in a scientific manner, and that the researchers were prejudiced in favor of the drug.

Although certainly even Dr. Pauling is anxious for a large-scale trial of vitamin C, the government and most research organizations simply don't have money for such projects; medicine has too many more pressing demands. A few years ago a congressman made a bid for research on the effects of honey on arthritis. His request was denied on the basis that although conclusions might be interesting, the paucity of evidence precluded investigation using public funds.

Another problem: It is difficult to judge results of treatment based on the pill user's testimony. For example, a person might notice that he has had fewer colds since taking vitamin C; however, he may also be taking better care of himself. Or his part of the country might be undergoing an unusually mild winter.

Iron supplements

"We're home, Mom," came the familiar cry at the kitchen door. "What's for lunch?"

"Go watch TV—I'm a little behind schedule," Margaret told her two youngsters, motioning to a newspaper in the corner for the deposit of muddy boots. Slapping two peanut butter sandwiches together and pouring two large glasses of milk, she hurried into the den. Dimly in the background she heard the blandishments of a frequently aired commercial for a product guaranteed to rejuvenate tired bodies and spirits. "That's what you need, Mom—I think you have tired blood," her oldest daughter remarked knowingly.

Maybe she's right, Margaret thought. Anyway, it wouldn't hurt to try. After all, maybe I'm so tired all the time because I'm anemic.

This lady's story illustrates the fact that, despite strict FDA regulations, the miracle mineral drugs—like vitamins—continue to hold their own in twentieth-century folk medicine (and "folks" are not all living on farms). Like vitamin pills, the advertised wonders of mineral products are supported essentially by the belief of the consumer.

The advertisements in a widely circulated health magazine called *Prevention* testify to the national obsession with wonder drugs, and to the fact that you can sell bathing suits to the eskimos if you convince them of the need. A few of the products promoted in this magazine: Vitamin E beauty cream; Sea-Algin from Giant Pacific Kelp, to help rid the system of "lead and fallout pollution"; "Super C-P," which blends vitamin C with "finest Wild Rose Hips, Citrus, Herbal Eucalyptus, in a compact oval 'power packed' tablet"; "Iron-Aid" tablets, for fitness and vitality—they make the blood red and thus help build and repair body tissues; Garlic Oil Perles, "Full natural essence of rich pungent oils captured in easy-to-take hermetically sealed capsules . . . seals in natural garlic aroma."

One of the oldest health products on the market is the iron supplement, guaranteed to make red blood redder and increase energy and endurance. Many people swear by their bottles of iron tonic, although the medical profession generally looks upon them with a jaundiced eye.

"Geritol is 15 per cent alcohol, that's why people sometimes feel better after drinking it," laughs Stuart C. Finch, M.D., head of the hematology department at Yale University School of Medicine. "Fatigue is certainly perhaps the most frequent complaint the doctor hears, but anemia is very rarely the cause, and iron supplements are simply a waste."

According to Dr. Finch, a recognized authority in the field of blood diseases, iron medications should not be given to anybody unless there is a specific medical reason. The most common cause of iron deficiency is excess bleeding, and if someone is bleeding, you should find out why, he explains.

"Excess iron intake can obscure the bleeding. In other words, the person medicating himself with iron pills may feel better and put off going to the doctor. Meanwhile, if he is bleeding from an intestinal tumor, the tumor is becoming more advanced. And even though short-term iron treatment may have no apparent side effects, we're not sure about the long run."

Dr. Finch is aggrieved by the high-powered promotion of products such as Geritol, "which has much less iron and is much more expensive than an iron tablet." Health products are particularly vulnerable to distorted presentation by advertisers, he points out, and the FDA should continue to wield a firm hand. Certain producers have been forced to modify their claims, but traps for the gullible still abound.

Dr. Finch believes that fatigue usually has an emotional basis unless it is the direct result of overwork. "Many people feel tired and in poor spirits a lot of the time and will try almost anything," he observes sympathetically. "Taking a pill or swallowing a spoonful of something makes them feel they are doing something positive for their condition."

Once a man has reached adulthood, the iron complement he carries will stay with him for the rest of his life, Dr. Finch explains. The body has no mechanism for excreting iron, thus the only way of losing it is through bleeding.

Women who are menstruating, pregnant, or nursing lose small

amounts of iron, but this loss is easily made up with iron supplements. In the case of menstruation, the blood loss is usually so small that no medication is necessary.

BIBLIOGRAPHY

"The Crash-Diet Craze," *Medical World News,* Apr. 27, 1973.

Family Fare: A Guide to Good Nutrition, U. S. Department of Agriculture, Home and Garden Bulletin No. 1, Washington, D.C., May 1970.

Flagler, J. M. "You and the Big Vitamin Battle," *Look,* June 1, 1971.

Keys, Ancel and Margaret. *Eat Well and Stay Well.* Doubleday, 1963.

Mayer, Jean. "Breakfast—Who Needs It?" *Family Health,* Sept. 1973.

———. "Shape Up and Slim Down," *Family Health,* Jan. 1974.

Pomeroy, Ruth Fairchild. "The New Nutrition: What Foods Really Keep You Healthy," *Redbook,* June 1972.

"The Prudent Diet: Vintage 1973," *Medical World News,* Aug. 10, 1973.

Spark, Richard F., M.D. "Fat Americans," *New York Times Magazine,* Jan. 6, 1974.

Waldo, Myra. *The International Encyclopedia of Cooking.* Macmillan, 1967.

7 DRUGS AND ALCOHOL: TIRED PEOPLE BEWARE

An unraveling of the mysteries of fatigue cannot proceed without pausing to analyze the twentieth-century's answer to every yawn, ache, or pain: drugs and alcohol.

Several years ago, parents, sociologists, psychiatrists, and practically everybody else were obsessed with the "degeneration" of today's drug-oriented youth, who reportedly drop acid or puff marijuana with little thought for the consequences.

Sixteen-year-old Johnny may smoke himself up the chimney on weekend parties with friends, but the family member who is most likely to be hooked—on legal drugs—is his mother.

The number of prescriptions for mood-altering drugs which doctors routinely fill out has climbed spectacularly in recent years to an annual total of some 225 million. One out of every three adult Americans acknowledges that he or she has used such drugs, and women pop twice as many pills as men. Typically, the heavy user is a woman between the ages of twenty-five and thirty-nine, with at least a high school diploma, who lives in a middle-class urban or suburban community.

The realization is beginning to grow that these legal drug takers, who may be renewing old prescriptions time after time without the doctor's knowledge, constitute a greater cause for concern in many cases than the lawbreakers. In fact, the National Commission on Marijuana and Drug Abuse reported in 1972 that the truth of the drug situation has been somewhat distorted by publicity.

In a national survey the Commission found that only 16 per cent of adults age eighteen and over and 14 per cent of youths twelve to seventeen years old had used marijuana at one time or another. Further, only thirteen million of the estimated twenty-six million who had smoked considered themselves "users."

Three per cent of the teen-agers and 4 per cent of adults had taken barbiturates for nonmedical reasons, and about the same numbers had tried stimulants, tranquilizers, or hallucinogens. Of the total group surveyed, 149,000 youths (0.6 per cent) and 1.8 million adults (1.3 per cent) had tried heroin at least once.

"While abuse of drugs by young people has received the attention of the mass media, the more significant issue, that of the ever-increasing use of legally prescribed drugs, has gone relatively unnoticed," notes Dr. Henry L. Lennard, associate professor of medical sociology at the University of California Medical Center, San Francisco.

Legal pill-popping can cause prolonged illness and can even lead to death, he points out. "The powerful chemicals damage kidneys and liver, destroy blood cells, injure brain tissue and nerve endings, affect eyesight, and profoundly depress blood pressure. Women taking the drugs often lose interest in sex; men may become impotent. Also, some psychoactive drugs are life-threatening when taken with other medications or with alcohol."

How did matters ever come to such a pass? Largely to blame is the attitude of contemporary society, which leads people to believe that gratifications should be instant and that pain or unpleasantness should not have to be endured. Advertisers hint that there is a pill for everything, and that we don't really have to cope with problems if we find the right product.

Doctors have also come under fire for being too ready to hand out a pill for almost any vague complaint. First, every physician is bombarded with advertisements for tranquilizers, sedatives, and stimulants, each manufacturer promising that his particular drug will bring about a miracle.

Rather than spend time with the patient drawing out his problems and perhaps referring him to a psychiatrist or social agency, the busy M.D. succumbs to the temptation to write out a prescription. That way, at least, the patient feels that something is being done for him.

Of course, psychoactive drugs have been of tremendous benefit to severly disturbed people—schizophrenics, paranoids, or manic depressives who are not equipped to face life by themselves and who can now function in normal society rather than wasting away in institutions.

Still, few of us are psychotics, and the wisdom of treating every emotional symptom as a manifestation of illness is questionable. Frequently a person suffers mental distress as a result of a social situation and not as a consequence of disturbed mental function. Yet more and more often, he is treated as if he, not his environment, were "sick."

What are barbiturates?

Back in the 1850s, modern chemistry provided man with his first chemical rather than botanical tension-reducing agent: the bromides. Bromides are poisonous, nonmetallic elements which, when combined with another element, produce a sedating effect on the consumer. Theoretically, bromides were used for the control of epilepsy and other spasmodic afflictions, but other uses were quickly found for them, and consumer demand began to swell enormously. Bromide abusers frequently developed the complications of delirium or psychosis.

Around 1930, the bromide problem began to ease, but only because other sedatives, primarily the barbiturates, were becoming available. The first barbiturate, Veronal, was followed quickly by pentobarbital, secobarbital, amobarbital, and other short-acting barbiturates, as well as by a long-acting drug like phenobarbital.

Only after a decade or so of use were the dependence-producing qualities of barbiturates recognized. Then, in the 1950s, a new class of drugs, the so-called minor tranquilizers, made their way to the marketplace.

These drugs have a barbiturate-like action and can produce both psychological and physical dependence; generally, however, they are held to be much less dangerous than their forebears. Their commercial names have become household words: Equanil, Miltown, Librium, Valium, etc.

Despite their bad reputation, barbiturates have a recognized place in medical treatment. They can help break the cycle of insomnia for some people, and for others they can restore normal sleep patterns.

Small doses of these drugs create drowsiness by depressing the function of those parts of the brain related to mental activities. For this reason, they are often prescribed for ulcer patients whose condition is related to excess worry and anxiety.

Large doses of certain barbiturates such as sodium pentothal are used as anesthetics for short-lasting operations. And phenobarbital is used to calm people in whom overactive thyroid glands produce abnormal motor activity.

Taken excessively over a long period of time, barbiturates are unquestionably harmful, although different people can withstand different amounts and the danger point is not easy to gauge. Many people take 0.2 grams, or two 1½-grain capsules, with no apparent ill effects. However, four times that amount taken for a few months will produce a dependency strong enough to give the user withdrawal symptoms similar to those of an alcoholic.

According to a Food and Drug Administration official, "From a purely physical viewpoint we feel that barbiturates are worse than narcotics. The habitual victim has difficulty thinking, cannot perform even simple calculations, loses the power to judge distances, becomes infantile, weeps easily and eventually has a desire for death."

Some fifteen hundred Americans die intentionally or accidentally every year from the acute form of barbiturate poisoning, the symptoms of which resemble to a large extent those of alcoholic intoxication. Older people and those in a weakened physical condition are particularly susceptible to the drugs, and people with liver or kidney disorders should not touch them.

Tragically, many people are not aware of when they reach the point of no return. First, people dosing themselves heavily may lose perception of the passage of time, replenishing themselves when they are still full of the drug. Also, barbiturates are absorbed slowly, and the pharmacologic effects are not felt immediately. Thus the user, who feels no change after a few pills, continues to take more and more until he is unconscious. If he has taken enough, he may never wake up.

In theory, barbiturates are available only with a prescription from the doctor, but the black market does a flourishing business. In addition, many "over the counter" products, such as antihistamines and antiemetics, have unpredictable or hypnotic effects.

According to the American Medical Association's Committee on Alcoholism and Addiction, many people swallow bottles of sedatives "to avoid reality, gain relief from tensions and anxieties. They take these drugs in lieu of or in addition to alcohol or opiates. Others follow the same procedure in search of paradoxical excitation and new thrills."

Drug dependence is a medical syndrome, the AMA points out, and almost always reflects some form of underlying mental disorder. The drug becomes "a symptom representation, a behavioristic reflection, of some form of psychological stress-functioning; an attempt to deal with or master some form of intrapsychic imbalance, conflict, or excitation."

Barbiturate dependence is particularly characteristic of "persons trying to deal with anxiety, guilt, aggression, inadequacy, depression, sexual urges, perversions, physical pain, and other expressions of psychoses, neuroses, and character disorders."

Essentially, there are four type of barbiturate abusers:

• Those seeking the sedative effects of the drug in order to deal with emotional distress;

• Those who have developed tolerance to the drugs after prolonged use and now need them, paradoxically, for exhilaration;

• Those who take the drugs to counteract the effects of stimulant drugs such as amphetamines;

• Alcoholics or narcotics users who also take barbiturates from time to time.

Kicking the sleeping-pill habit

Most habitual sleeping-pill poppers are in none of the foregoing categories; they take sleeping pills because they can't get to sleep at night. Some sleeping pills are so weak that their main effect is psychological; the pill swallower believes that the pill will help him fall asleep, and therefore it does. This is called the placebo effect.

Prolonged use of these pills, however, builds up a tolerance to them, and the user needs more and more to put him to sleep. Not only is addiction to sedatives dangerous to health, it can wreak havoc on normal sleep patterns, thus frustrating the original intention.

Two brain chemicals, serotonin and norepinephrine, are both altered by sleeping pills. Serotonin plays a role in helping us fall asleep and reach delta sleep, while norepinephrine is believed to mediate the dreaming stage. Distortion of any phase of sleep will produce predictably unhappy results (see Chapter 3).

Why do people continue taking sleeping pills against everybody's advice and against their own common sense? First, because of the "dream rebound" phenomenon that strikes on the first pill-less night. Because REM sleep has been depressed during the time the person was using sedatives regularly, it now demands a major share of sleep time.

In other words, the first night that the pill user decides to forego his security blanket, he will find himself dreaming constantly, as if his unconscious life were a double-feature movie, and he will spend the whole night tossing and turning. These dreams often take the form of hair-raising nightmares or anxiety dreams.

If a habitual user suddenly stops taking his pills, he may also suffer such serious effects as convulsions, delirium, hallucinations, or a rise in blood pressure. For this reason the intelligent physician will guide his patient through a progressive recovery and not ask him to go "cold turkey."

Dr. Peter Hauri, director of the Dartmouth Sleep Laboratory, issues his patients a list of progressive relaxation exercises that he can do at home, the object being to relax his muscles so that he is not so terrified of the thought of going to sleep without pills.

He also uses biofeedback techniques wherein some parameter of the patient's body—his brain waves, muscle tension, or some other area not usually controlled—is displayed to the patient on electronic equipment. Thus the patient can appreciate what conscious or unconscious moves increase his muscle tension, for instance.

"Only when the patient becomes adept either at relaxation exercises or some sort of biofeedback can he start thinking about reducing his pill intake," says Dr. Hauri. "In addition to gradually reducing the pills, we also do our best to control the REM rebound, reintroducing dream sleep in such a way that the patient will not get too anxious or upset."

The habitual sleeping-pill user is in particular trouble if he is also a drinker, because the combination of barbiturates and alcohol can often be fatal, even if the amount of the individual substances is not great. Many cases are on record of people who died through ignorance of these biochemical facts.

In addition, we are all subject to variations in our tolerance of particular substances. For instance, drugs can produce much stronger effects in a person who is dog-tired, or who has not eaten for a long time. If a person taking sleeping pills is also taking other medications, he may suffer unforeseen ill effects from the combination of the two.

Are there any drugs which can be safely used as sleep-inducers? Even the mildest medications can become the basis of an undesirable psychological addiction. However, since the clamor for sleeping pills is not about to die down, researchers have been looking hard for a substance which will sedate without the complications.

The phenothiazines such as chlorpromazine are not addictive and present few serious overdose problems, Dr. James L. Claghorn, associate professor of psychiatry, University of Texas School of Medicine at Houston, points out.

"Many people can achieve a satisfactory night's sleep without morning hangovers with proper doses of these major tranquilizers. You have to consider the side effects, but in patients with severe insomnia, they may be well worth trying."

Antihistamines, particularly diphenhydramine HC1 (Benadryl), can be used very successfully as a nighttime sedative, he adds. "Some patients experience morning hangovers, but most can take it quite comfortably. Benadryl is a safe and easily managed sedative."

What are amphetamines?

Every year drug companies pour close to ten billion amphetamines into the eager hands of waiting Americans. Some 50 per cent of these pills, best known by the brand names Dexedrine and Benzedrine, wind up on the black market, where they are bought not for medical use, but as a quick route to a "high."

Both amphetamine and methamphetamine, the main stimulant drugs, were synthesized in the 1920s as part of the search for a substitute for ephedrine. Pharmacologically, these drugs are sympathomimetic amines which are closely related to adrenalin and ephedrine, but with a much stronger stimulating effect on the central nervous system.

In the beginning, amphetamines were given to people who had to perform tiring tasks for extended periods or who had to stay awake for long stretches. Many doctors who now caution their patients against the horrors of amphetamine abuse were not above swallowing one now and again during their harried medical school and internship days.

Gradually, more legitimate medical uses were found for these drugs, including treatment of sleeping sickness, muscle disorders, and mild depression. But before amphetamine-containing diet pills were taken off the market recently, the most popular medical use for amphetamines was undoubtedly for weight control.

For the embattled dieter, a diet pill (or anorexiant) offered two great advantages: It took away his appetite and gave him a jazzed-up feeling of well-being. Many people became hooked on the pills and yet did not lose weight in the long run.

Although amphetamines are not physically addictive, habitual users often become psychologically hooked to the point where they cannot get through a day without them. Because the body develops a tolerance to these pills, more and more are needed to achieve the same effect.

Often a person becomes dependent quite without intending to. An overweight teen-ager named Gretchen recalls how her pleas and lamentations finally led her doctor to prescribe appetite depressants, and how she did lose weight initially, but gradually built up a tolerance to the drugs. On days when she expected to be faced with

groaning tables of food—Thanksgiving, birthdays, evenings out—
she would down two or three pills.

When the doctor noticed that Gretchen's requests for refills were
coming fast on the heels of one another, he called a halt. Gretchen
decided to give life-without-pills a try; however, she suffered a rebound depression that sent her to another doctor who would prescribe the pills.

Gretchen had grown happily used to the slight mood elevation
the pills provided and couldn't face the crash period that followed
abandoning them, although she had been told that her body would
soon readjust to the lack of stimulation.

Eventually her consumption reached the level where in order to
get to sleep at night, she needed a barbiturate to calm her down.
Thus the vicious circle began to roll: uppers to get her through the
day, downers to put her to sleep.

Amphetamine abuse is a mushrooming evil in this country as well
as in Great Britain, Japan, Canada, Sweden, and other countries.
The problem is twofold: People don't care what they take as long as
they think it's helping them, and many physicians give too little consideration to the dependence-producing properties of the drug. Consequently they hand out prescriptions almost on demand, and before
they know it, their patient is in trouble.

The road to euphoria and back

Amphetamine users constitute a very mixed bunch, from the college
student or truck driver who pops an occasional pill to keep himself
awake for the long haul, to the speed freak who injects vast amounts
of the drug into his veins. Many of the latter have been found dead
with a needle in their arms. Death can result from cardiac arrest,
infection, or a suicide attempt.

Alcoholics and other drug abusers may take amphetamines as
antidotes for alcohol or hypnotic drugs, and also to give their
psyches a boost when depression threatens. But perhaps the most
common abuser comes from the ranks of dieters, women in particular, who originally got hold of the pills for weight reduction and now
find they cannot get along without their 10 mg of sustained-release
dextroamphetamine each morning.

Included among the amphetamine-type drugs are dl-amphetamine

(Benzedrine), dextroamphetamine (Dexedrine), methamphetamine (Desoxyn), phenmetrazine (Preludin), methylphenidate (Ritalin), diethylpropion (Tenuate), and pipradol (Meratran). Some act directly, others indirectly, on the adrenergic nerve endings, but all have some effect on the central nervous system.

People will react differently to these drugs according to how long they have been using them and how much they are taking. Small oral doses (5 to 10 mg) of dextroamphetamine, for example, usually causes only mild mood elevation, slight nervousness, loss of appetite, insomnia, relief of fatigue, and a euphoric sense of enhanced physical and mental efficiency.

The psychological high lasts for only a few hours, however, and is often succeeded by a letdown period during which the user feels depressed and tired. Once a person is hooked on the pills, he has to take increasing doses in order to achieve the same initial effects on mood and appetite.

Occasionally, amphetamine abuse can result in acute paranoid psychosis. In this state the victim may undergo both auditory and visual hallucinations, even though he is clear-minded, and he exhibits many of the characteristics of a paranoid state. He may even start attacking people.

Generally, the psychotic symptoms will disappear within two weeks after the drug is withdrawn, but doctors stress that without supportive aftercare, usually including psychotherapy, many people will return to their old habits and possibly wind up in the hospital. Occasional patients remain permanently psychotic.

A British expert, Dr. Philip H. Connell of the Maudsley Hospital in London, is particularly careful to look for signs of amphetamine abuse in the following types:

· Teen-agers who express feelings of aggression toward their parents, especially the mother, and who are notorious for rapid changes of mood and for staying out late;

· Paranoid psychotics;

· Tired housewives, or obese people, with anxiety and some depression;

· Physicians, pharmacists, nurses, or musicians who come to the doctor with signs of tension anxiety or depression.

"In general practice, however, there are other types of patients who must be suspected to be amphetamine-dependent," Dr. Connell stresses. "These include the patient who asks specifically for the drug, who has lost the pills, or dropped them down the toilet, or says that the children have thrown them away; the obese patient who in spite of not losing weight still insists on having the amphetamine."

Many people are not aware that amphetamines are not a magic source of extra mental or physical energy; rather, they only push the user to burn up his own resources, sometimes to a point of exhaustion. Unfortunately, the chronic amphetamine user is not able to assess his own ability to perform. This fact has led to a number of automobile fatalities, in addition to less lethal accidents.

According to the AMA's Committee on Alcoholism and Addiction, abuse of the amphetamine-type drugs almost invariably reflects some underlying form of psychopathology. "Amphetamine dependence is a medical syndrome; a symptom complex that usually reflects some form of psychological and behavioristic disorder," the Committee points out.

"The stimulant is commonly used as an 'adjustive' mechanism to help the person 'deal' with problems of living and emotional difficulties. Abuse constitutes a 'reaching out' for something without which the patient feels relatively helpless, and there is a continuum between what constitutes ill-advised 'self-medication' and full abuse."

Reaching for recovery

Like other drug abusers, the amphetamine user is very vulnerable to relapse, no matter how good his intentions. Nevertheless, many cases of complete recovery are on record, particularly among people who first started taking the drug as a form of social experimentation.

For people who have been injecting themselves with amphetamines over a long period, the "crash" is a nightmare, literally and metaphorically. The person will sleep for as long as two days, often enduring severe nightmares, and will awaken ravenously hungry. The paranoid psychosis usually clears quickly, but the victim then becomes apathetic and depressed, often to the point where he goes right back on the drug treadmill.

For the moderate user, all measurable traces of amphetamine should disappear from the body within a week, but he does not get off scot-free. For example, if the pills are masking an underlying depression, the depression will emerge when the user stops taking the drug. Also, if the amphetamines were used mainly as an antidote to chronic fatigue, a two- or three-day period of intense tiredness often follows.

For the severe abuser, who is frequently taking barbiturates as well, the hospital is the safest place for withdrawal. Many people can be taken safely off amphetamines without entering the hospital, however, if the doctor is thoroughly aware of past and present drug history and if he is certain the patient is not secretly resupplying himself.

As with other forms of drug abuse, withdrawal is only the beginning of the treatment process. As the AMA report points out, "The physician should be prepared to maintain contact with the patient and be available for specific psychotherapy, or at least supportive help, for a long period. If such support is not forthcoming, the patient will probably relapse and renew his drug dependence."

Every amphetamine abuser should undergo complete medical, psychological, and social assessment, with particular attention to any problems relating to job, marriage, or family. If possible, members of the patient's family should be seen periodically. Psychiatric referrals should be made wherever feasible.

Unfortunately, the road to recovery is uphill, and despite honest intentions on the part of both users and those treating them, the record has not been too encouraging. For example, in 1972 psychiatrists at Massachusetts General Hospital in Boston reported on a series of two hundred and eight patients between the ages of thirteen and thirty who had abused amphetamines, barbiturates, and hallucinogens. During an eighteen-month period when they were treated as hospital outpatients, only one of the entire group returned for regularly scheduled therapy. Of eighty-three patients to whom continuing psychiatric care was offered, eight returned for a single visit, and only one followed through with the recommended treatment.

Analyzing these discouraging results, Lieutenant Commander William H. Anderson, MC, USN, the naval psychiatrist who headed the study, made this comment: "For most of these drug abusers the abstinent state has nothing to offer them except real or imagined grim life circumstances. Drugs offer an immediate release from frustrations; a therapist cannot compete with this."

Traditional psychotherapy offers no immediate solutions, he acknowledges. "This fact probably comes closer to the actuality of our failure to deal with drug abuse. We do not have the tools or the knowledge to offer a better alternative."

Alcohol and fatigue

For the man or woman who has found a comfortable and necessary place for alcohol in his or her life, the first instinct after a particularly tiring day is often to reach for a tray of ice cubes and open the liquor cabinet. A stiff drink seems just what the doctor ordered to revive spirits and relax tension.

Moderate amounts of alcohol are stimulating and pleasant, producing a temporary sense of warmth and well-being. But alcohol can act as a drug, a beverage, or a poison, depending on how it is used.

When a person takes a drink, the blood vessels of his skin dilate, bringing an increased flow of warm blood to the skin surfaces. This process results in a cooling off of the blood and an eventual drop in body temperature.

The most impressive physiologic effects of alcohol are upon the central nervous system. While the first drink or two makes a person feel relaxed and cheerful, a large amount inevitably acts as a depressant. Drinking events usually feature at least one guest who is the life of the party at 9 P.M., but by midnight is sitting in an armchair staring morosely into his drink. If he is the type in whom alcohol brings out anxiety, suspicion, and distrust, he may be locked in argument with his host.

Alcohol acts as an anesthetic upon the cerebral cortex, the area of the brain which controls behavior. This explains the characteristic "uninhibited" behavior of the person who is flying high, and who is now ready to tell his boss that he needs more money, his wife that she should lose weight, or his son that he loves him.

As the drinking continues, he becomes less and less aware of his environment, both internal and external. He may not notice that he has burned his finger with a match, and he may not think about the dangers of driving home later that night. Eventually, he may begin to stagger about the room, dropping things and slurring his words.

Nutritionally speaking, alcohol is fairly useless: it is quickly burnt up, cannot be stored, and has little food value. It does pack a number of calories. Heavy drinkers are often overweight and poorly nourished.

The consequences of a one-night binge may include nausea, vomiting, and diarrhea. Prolonged and excessive use of alcohol takes a heavy toll on the gastrointestinal tract and may lead to chronic gastritis, ulceration, and hemorrhage. Extremely heavy drinking can also damage the liver, the kidneys, and other organs.

Where does alcoholism begin?

For years, scientists have been trying to define alcoholism, which is now recognized as a medical disease. Some people have argued that the causes are biological, and that a person is born with the tendency to become an alcoholic. Others have maintained that the causes are environmental, and that alcoholism is a learned behavior pattern.

According to Dr. Frank Seixas, medical director of the National Council on Alcoholism, no one single triggering factor has yet been identified. "We have found families where the women are prone to depression and the men to alcoholism," he reports. "And other investigators have found a connection between color vision defects, blood clotting defects, and alcoholism. These findings, however, are not yet conclusive."

In the past, and still in many hospitals today, the alcoholic has been treated as the stepchild of the medical ward; frequently he is admitted under a false diagnosis, such as ulcer disease. Part of the problem is that physicians become frustrated in treating alcoholics, who often fall from grace and are back in the office to start all over. Also, medical schools tend to skip lightly over alcoholism, and as a result too many doctors share the common belief that it is a self-induced disease.

The American Medical Association defines alcoholism as "an illness characterized by preoccupation with alcohol and loss of control over its consumption such as to lead usually to intoxication if drinking is begun; by chronicity; by progression; and by tendency toward relapse. It is typically associated with physical disability and impaired emotional, occupational, and/or social adjustments as a direct consequence of persistent and excessive use of alcohol."

In other words, alcoholism is a type of drug dependence which usually interferes seriously with the patient's total health and his relationship to his environment.

Not every alcoholic is lolling in the doorsteps of Skid Row, needless to say. Many men and women who hold well-paid and responsible positions are attending meetings of Alcoholics Anonymous twice a week in an effort to cure themselves, while others are nervously praying that their "weakness" will not be discovered.

Non-working women in particular, for a variety of social reasons, tend to be secret drinkers who nip away at the sherry bottle during the day, then join their husbands in the evening for a "first" cocktail.

Because people's tolerance for alcohol varies widely, it is often difficult to draw the line between heavy drinking and alcoholism. Dr. Harris Isbell, professor of medicine and pharmacology at the University of Kentucky College of Medicine, puts it this way:

"The incipient alcoholic simply drinks more than his peers. The wine drinker is no longer content with a glass at meals but drinks an entire bottle. Such drinking may persist for years, but gradually the pattern becomes exaggerated."

Alcoholics continue to drink after the party is over and to the point of stupor, he observes. Some go on binges of two or three days' duration, while others start drinking alone at night.

Eventually, "drinking becomes daily rather than periodic. The person is 'hung over' each morning and begins to drink to alleviate the hangover, presaging the development of addiction. Personality deterioration sets in. The alcoholic becomes resentful of advice, blames his drinking on others, is forgetful, unreliable, and quarrelsome."

There is, however, no well-defined "alcoholic personality." An alcoholic may drink steadily day after day, or he may have short periods of abstinence, followed by colossal binges.

Curing the disease

For the alcoholic in an acute state of intoxication and who may be in a stupor or coma, the only place is the hospital. First, while he is suffering delirium tremens, he is dangerous to himself. Losing all sense of time, space, and surroundings, he endures terrifying visual hallucinations and may harm himself trying to escape from them. The DTs last for three to seven days, and the patient can end up in the morgue if he is not properly cared for meanwhile.

Estimates vary, but many experts peg the number of alcoholic Americans at 4.5 million. Although the figure is staggering, the total picture is far from grim. According to Dr. Seixas, even without treatment, 5 to 10 per cent of alcoholics will improve to the point where they can lead normal lives.

"Alcoholics Anonymous controls alcoholism in another 20 per cent, and 30 per cent of the people treated at a clinic get better," he relates. "And by 'get better' I mean abstinence or a very marked social improvement. Also, 80 per cent of persons taking part in labor-management programs in alcoholism improve."

In fact, any kind of intervention has a positive influence on the alcoholic mortality rate, which is extremely high. Alcoholics also commit suicide at a rate fifty-eight times greater than that of the general population.

Rehabilitation of the alcoholic rests on three cornerstones: group therapy, disulfiram (Antabuse), and Alcoholics Anonymous.

Group therapy sessions have been led successfully by a number of professionals, including social service workers, psychologists, and psychiatrists, in addition to recovered alcoholics who have become AA counselors.

"Family therapy has also been enormously helpful," Dr. Seixas reports. "During the five to fifteen years that it may take for alcoholism to develop, there are a lot of interactions that take place and a lot of changes in the equilibrium between the two partners to the marriage and the children. The spouse needs treatment badly because of the disordered pattern of life."

Antabuse is a drug which blocks the oxidation of alcohol; a person who drinks after he has swallowed the drug will suffer nausea, vomiting, vasodilation, and even cardiovascular collapse. Although Antabuse alone is not enough, many people find that with half a tablet once a day, they can withstand sobriety for much longer periods than normally.

"It is particularly valuable for someone who is committed to sobriety but who finds that in our culture, with a bar on every corner, he really has a hard time remaining sober through the day without some kind of insurance policy," Dr. Seixas points out.

Among the many organizations dedicated to helping the alcoholic, Alcoholics Anonymous has achieved the widest acclaim. AA groups are made up of men and women who have overcome their own addiction and who can supply the sympathy and understanding which the alcoholic needs in order to launch himself on the road to recovery.

Another undocumented but significant factor in the more hopeful outlook for the alcoholic is the change in attitude which society has undergone in recent years. Not long ago, the alcoholic was looked upon with amusement and scorn, with a judgmental and moralizing eye. Today, people are beginning to understand that alcoholism, like cancer, is a disease, and that our job is not to punish, but to help.

BIBLIOGRAPHY

"Alcoholism—A Call for Early Detection, Aggressive Management," *Medical World News,* Oct. 13, 1972.

American Medical Association. *Manual on Alcoholism,* 1973.

AMA Committee on Alcoholism and Addiction. "Dependence on Amphetamines and Other Stimulant Drugs," *JAMA,* Sept. 19, 1966.

————. "Dependence on Barbiturates and Other Sedative Drugs," *JAMA,* Aug. 23, 1965.

Anderson, William H., Lt. Cdr. "Failure of Outpatient Treatment of Drug Abuse," *American Journal of Psychiatry,* June 1972.

Beeson, Paul B., M.D., and McDermott, Walsh, M.D., eds. *Cecil-Loeb Textbook of Medicine.* Saunders, 1971.

Berg, Roland H. "The Over-Medicated Woman," *McCall's,* Sept. 1971.

Connell, Philip H., M.D. "Clinical Manifestations and Treatment of Amphetamine Type of Dependence," *JAMA,* May 23, 1966.

Deming, Richard. *Sleep, Our Unknown Life.* Nelson, 1972.

Fishbein, Morris, M.D., ed. *The Modern Family Health Guide.* Doubleday, 1967.

Freedman, Daniel X., M.D. "The President's Commission on Drug Abuse," *Psychiatry*. McGraw-Hill, 1973.

————. "Office Therapy for Anxiety/Depression," *Patient Care*, Aug. 1, 1973.

Scarf, Maggie. "Oh, for a Decent Night's Sleep!" *New York Times Magazine*, Oct. 21, 1973.

8 THE STATE OF YOUR HEALTH

How long has it been since you've seen a doctor? Many people do not bother with an annual physical examination as long as they are feeling all right. Yet fatigue is a symptom of a wide spectrum of medical conditions.

Dr. James B. Donaldson, professor of medicine at Temple University in Philadelphia, asks the following seven questions of patients who come to him complaining of fatigue:

- What do you mean by fatigue?
- How long has this condition existed?
- Did it come about suddenly, or has it mushroomed over a period of time?
- Do you sleep well? How do you feel in the morning?
- Have you lost weight recently, and if so, how much?
- How is your appetite?
- Are you under any particular emotional strain?

This history-taking, he stresses, is the most important element in the diagnosis; unless the doctor listens closely to the patient's story first, he might as well forget the physical examination and laboratory tests.

If a physician has examined you recently, a complete workup may not be necessary unless there has been a change in your health picture. If this is the first visit to a new doctor, you will probably want him to examine you thoroughly.

Generally, the older the patient, the more likely his fatigue has an organic basis such as diabetes, thyroid abnormalities, or a blood disease such as anemia. In a younger patient, fatigue may result from poor nutrition, obesity, or perhaps an incipient illness such as mononucleosis.

What are the possible physical causes of fatigue?

Diabetes mellitus

The essential factor in this metabolic disorder is insufficiency of insulin, a hormone which is secreted in the pancreas. When a person lacks insulin, his body is unable to transform the sugar from carbohydrate foods into glycogen, the substance which the muscles draw on for fuel. The sugar then remains in the diabetic's blood and is excreted in his urine, unavailable to the tissues and organs needing it.

Since 1921, when synthetic insulin was discovered, the lives of diabetics have been extended in many cases to normal expectancy. Before that, these people generally died before the age of five.

Diabetes in its fully developed form is marked by weakness, lethargy, loss of weight, and failure to grow. A blood sugar test taken in the doctor's office will immediately establish the condition. The diabetic who does not know of his illness and is taking vitamins or amphetamines for his symptoms is inviting trouble; these drugs can often make the disease worse.

Obesity tends to aggravate diabetes. Also, people who are grossly overweight often become diabetic even though they were quite normal before. Babies are rarely diabetic; susceptibility increases with age. In the general population, about 1.5 per cent will be diabetics, although this figure rises as high as 10 per cent in people over age sixty. Women are more often the victims before the age of menopause, and the more children a woman has, the more likely she is to develop the disease.

The origins of diabetes are uncertain, but many investigators believe it is related to some disorder in the central nervous system that involves the area of the brain associated with the pituitary gland. While diabetes tends to run in families, it is a recessive characteristic; in other words, unless reinforced by the addition of new diabetes-prone members, a family will tend to breed it out. Thanks to the discovery of insulin, diabetes today is less of a health threat than a major infection. Insulin does not cure the condition, however, and the diabetic must observe many precautions all of his life, particularly about the food he eats.

Mononucleosis

Infectious mononucleosis, or "kissing disease," is a virus infection which causes a swelling of the lymph glands and changes in the white blood cells. Most often it strikes people between the ages of ten and thirty-five, among whom the virus is often passed in saliva during kissing. Usually mono lasts from three to six weeks.

Fatigue is often the earliest symptom of the disease. In addition, the victim will be feverish, his glands swollen, and his throat red and sore with patches or sheets of grayish discharge. Mono may also cause headaches and sometimes a loss of appetite. Occasionally a discolored rash will erupt on the skin: other times liver disfunction produces a jaundiced color. Occasionally, the mono sufferer may have no symptoms at all.

Only a few years ago many researchers believed that mono was a stress illness typical of college students, brought on by prolonged pressure, anxiety, and depression. Now the general opinion is that while a person in good physical condition is less likely to develop mono, the disease is caused by transmission of the EB virus, not by studying too hard.

Because mono mimics many other illnesses, from tonsilitis to serious blood disorders, physicians who seldom see the disease may have difficulty identifying it. Today, it is easy to confirm the diagnosis by sending a sample of the patient's blood to a lab.

The best treatment for mono is to rest, usually in bed, until all fever or acute symptoms have subsided. Because the disease is virally induced, antibiotics are ineffective and may even produce an allergic reaction. Sore throats demand hot salt gargles, and special diets are usually prescribed when the patient has jaundice.

Mono is only mildly contagious, and there is no need for the patient to be isolated. In addition to kissing, it can be transmitted by sharing the same glass or eating from the same piece of fruit.

Hepatitis

This virally-caused infection is perhaps the most frequently encountered disorder of the liver. At least two forms are known: infectious hepatitis, which is transmitted in much the same manner as a cold, and serum hepatitis, which enters the body directly via the blood, for example during a blood transfusion or during injection with an unsterilized needle.

Frequently, infectious hepatitis is spread through water or food which has been contaminated. Jaundice is the most noticeable symptom; however, the victim may also suffer fatigue, loss of appetite, fever and chills, backache, heartburn, nausea, vomiting, and diarrhea. As with mononucleosis, the foundation of treatment is bed rest. Most doctors will also prescribe a high-protein, high-carbohydrate diet with few fats.

Sometimes a person who has had infectious hepatitis will develop chronic low-grade liver insufficiency, but most people will be cured completely within time.

Serum hepatitis develops more gradually, with similar symptoms, but the condition is much more serious than the infectious form. It may take many months for the victim to recover, and he may be left with a badly damaged liver.

Hypothyroidism

When a person's thyroid gland is sluggish, he becomes mentally as well as physically lethargic. A child born with this deficiency will be retarded both physically and mentally, and will become a dwarf of low mental capacity, termed a cretin.

Adults can develop hypothyroidism spontaneously, leading to what is called myxedema. Sometimes this condition is the consequence of surgery or other treatment for hyperthyroidism, when the remaining amount of thyroid tissue is not enough for the body's needs.

Recently, lowered thyroid activity has been implicated in a number of symptoms: poor equilibrium, muscle aches and weakness, some hearing disturbances, and nervous-system changes leading to burning and prickling sensations, mental depression, memory loss, and difficulties in concentrating.

Various means are used to detect low thyroid, including a basal metabolism test and a protein-bound iodine and radioactive-iodine uptake test. Thyroid extract pills are generally successful in correcting the condition.

Coronary thrombosis

Many people who have suffered a heart attack admit later to having felt tired out for days or weeks before the event. Some become so used to their symptoms that they accept them as a normal state of affairs.

Coronary thrombosis is a rather loose term used to describe the blocking of an artery of the heart. Usually, the victim's circulation has slowed or his arterial walls have thickened to a point where a clot of blood forms within the heart or blood vessels.

This process may be a rapid one, or it may develop over a long period of time. When the occlusion occurs rapidly, the patient may die suddenly if the blocking involves a large artery or occurs in an already damaged heart muscle. However, if the obstruction occurs in a smaller branch of the coronary arteries, chances for recovery are good.

The primary cause of coronary artery disease is not known, but in most cases thrombosis occurs in a coronary artery that has become thickened and hardened, leading to clot formation that prevents blood from flowing to the heart muscle.

The condition rarely develops in people younger than forty, and men are struck more often than women. Frequently, the victims are active and high-strung, or they are under severe mental and emotional stress. Conditions which often lead to heart attack include angina pectoris (chest pain), high blood pressure, arteriosclerosis (hardening of the arteries), nephritis (kidney inflammation), and syphilis.

The history of a heart attack is usually as follows: The victim is suddenly seized with excruciating pain over the heart, which spreads rapidly all over the front of the chest and sometimes down over the abdomen. Often he will collapse.

Although a person can live a long time after a heart attack, the crisis must be taken seriously, and most physicians will counsel from three to six weeks of bed rest before the resumption of normal activities.

Hypoglycemia

Hypoglycemia exists when a person's body is producing too much insulin and the blood sugar (glucose) falls to an abnormally low level. Diabetics are victims of the opposite condition—hyperglycemia, where the body tries to correct for a chronic lack of insulin by pouring excess sugar into the urine.

Hypoglycemia can be a symptom of several conditions: malnutrition, malabsorption (improper utilization of foods), a tumor, adrenocortical or pituitary failure, liver necrosis, Reye's syndrome. Sometimes it is the precursor to diabetes, other times it signifies a hereditary fructose intolerance. Some people who have undergone a gastrectomy (removal of all or part of the stomach) become hypoglycemic.

A physician will suspect hypoglycemia in a person who suddenly goes into a coma or who suffers periodic episodes of confusion, convulsions, weakness, fatigue, or inappropriate hunger. Treatment includes glucose infusions and frequently a change of diet.

Anemia

Anemia, which occurs when the concentration of hemoglobin in the blood falls below a normal level, is characterized by a general feeling of tiredness. The condition can be caused simply by loss of blood, such as from an injury or from internal hemorrhaging, or it may result from a destruction of cells or from inadequate formation of cells.

When anemia is caused by blood loss, a doctor will first stop the bleeding, then prescribe rest and proper diet, including iron and protein for building cells.

In anemia caused by abnormal breakdown of red blood cells, called hemolytic anemia, hemoglobin is released at a much greater rate than it can be replaced. Frequently, the manufacture of bile pigments is excessive, and the victim develops the yellowish skin characteristic of hemolytic jaundice. Hemolytic anemia can be a disease one is born with, such as sickle cell anemia, or it may be the result of illness.

Nutritional anemias occur when a person is not getting enough of a particular substance, usually iron, and consequently his body cannot produce enough hemoglobin. A diet deficient in iron may cause fainting spells and difficulty in breathing as well as weakness and fatigue. Proper food and rest usually cure the condition.

When a pregnant woman becomes anemic, it is usually because of the increased demands being made on her circulatory system, which must carry food, oxygen, and waste products for two human beings. If her diet is poor or if she is vomiting a lot, the problem will be made worse, and the doctor will probably prescribe iron and protein supplements.

Defective bone formation can produce bone marrow deficiency disease, probably the most serious form of anemia. To mature properly, the red cells in the body must have a substance from the liver called the growth or maturation factor, which is closely related to vitamin B_{12}. To absorb this vitamin the body uses a substance found in normal gastric juice called the intrinsic factor.

In some anemias, the intrinsic factor is absent, while in others the maturation factor is in scant supply. Pernicious anemia, for example, is characterized by the disappearance of this intrinsic factor as well as of hydrochloric acid in the gastric juice. Pernicious anemia and several other types respond well to liver injections alone or combined with vitamin B_{12}.

Influenza

Influenza is one of many well-known diseases caused by viruses and including the common cold, measles, German measles, chicken pox, mumps, rabies, poliomyelitis, encephalitis, and smallpox. These diseases are transmitted in a variety of ways, sometimes by direct contact, sometimes by airborne droplets of nasal and salivary secretions.

Popularly known as the flu or grippe, influenza is a highly contagious disease which usually appears in the winter in epidemic form. It spreads with great rapidity but usually runs a definite course within a short period of time. The flu is rarely serious in itself, but the victim tends to be more susceptible from then on to secondary infections of the lungs which may become serious.

Most people will recover quickly after a bout of one to five days, although they are often left with a feeling of weakness and general depression. No one has found a specific cure for the flu; at the moment, the best treatment is to go to bed as soon as you think you have it and stay there until you feel completely recovered. While running a fever, drink large quantities of liquids.

Hemorrhoids

A person with hemorrhoids may find that the little bit of blood he loses each night is enough to weaken him the next morning.

Hemorrhoids, or piles, are actually swollen varicose veins that appear at the lower end of the bowel on the margin of the anus. External hemorrhoids may produce little more than itching or a feeling of tightness during a bowel movement. Internal hemorrhoids sometimes become infected and inflamed, leading to clotting or thrombosis. They may also protrude and bleed if scratched or broken.

Medicine has devised several methods of treating hemorrhoids; surgery is a radical but effective one. For many people, the answer is to correct the condition that brought on the hemorrhoids in the first place, including extremely sedentary habits, overweight, or chronic constipation.

Obesity

Obviously, a person who is lugging around a great mass of flesh is going to collapse into an armchair a lot sooner than his thin friends. Often a reduction of a mere fifteen pounds or so will make a considerable difference in his energy reserves.

Many physicians feel that a person is at a medical danger point when he is 20 per cent above his normal weight, although this point is argued. Experts generally agree, however, that most people are fat for one reason: They eat too much. Few and far between are the fatties who can blame their woes on organic disease or on a pituitary or thyroid disturbance. Some women become obese as a result of changes in the secretions of their sex organs during pregnancy or menopause.

In general, we have only ourselves to blame for our bulk, but it is true that some families, and even certain races, tend to produce fat members. Food which is not used for energy is stored as fat and deposited in various parts of the body, particularly the hips, stomach, breasts, and buttocks. Fat may also be stored around the heart and liver, interfering with the normal functioning of these organs.

In addition to tiring quickly, fat people are often short of breath. Their legs and feet are subjected to undue strain, which predisposes them to flat feet and to osteoarthritis of the knees and lower back.

Fat people are also more prone to heart disturbances, diseases of the pancreas, kidneys, and gall bladder, and diabetes. The extremely obese die earlier of natural causes, and they are also more likely to die of complications on the operating table.

Visual fatigue

A person who is using his eyes a great deal and who notices unaccustomed fatigue may simply need glasses. Seeing is a muscular function, and some visual tasks require a great deal of action from the tiny sets of muscles within the eye. For example, a job that demands frequent shifts, from examining fine print to looking at objects in the distance, would be wearing to the eye muscles. A proper pair of glasses allows a person to use his eyes for longer periods without straining.

People's "eyes get tried" not only when their eye muscles are overtaxed, but when they don't enjoy what they are reading. This fatigue is akin to the "mental fatigue" one suffers when performing a difficult or demanding intellectual task, such as memorizing a list of a hundred Chinese words.

Menstruation

Many women can tie their energy-fatigue cycle directly to their menstrual cycle. Theoretically, a woman menstruates every twenty-eight days for a period of four to five days; however, three-week or five-week cycles are common, and a number of women are consistently irregular.

Almost every menstruating woman will suffer some degree of premenstrual tension before her period, often taking the form of fatigue and depression. Although it is not known exactly why this happens, generally the phenomenon is attributed to a change in the balance between two hormones, estrogen and progesterone.

About a week before the onset of menstruation, the hormonal shift causes a woman's body and brain to retain water and swell; apparently, the brain swelling provides the physiologic basis for the "premenstrual blues." There is really little to be done for this condition except to wait it out and perhaps take a tranquilizer.

Fatigue is also common to women who are actually menstruating, although the amount of blood they lose is usually very small. Violent sports or other activities are generally not recommended during the days of heavy flow, but most twentieth-century women do not find it necessary to restrict their daily routine to any great extent.

There are two abnormal conditions which may indeed cause excessive fatigue: menorrhagia, or the loss of an excessive amount of blood during menstruation, and metrorrhagia, the excessive flow of blood between periods. Naturally, any woman with either condition should see a physician at once.

Menopause

Like menstruation, menopause is a normal event in a woman's life cycle which may be accompanied by excessive fatigue. Menopause, or the cessation of menstruation, usually takes place when a woman is between the ages of forty-five and fifty-five. At this time her ovaries (the female sex glands) become relatively inactive, and other changes occur in her body.

Some women sail through menopause without the slightest signs of discomfort. For others, it is an uncomfortable and difficult period which may last as long as four years.

The most common physical symptom is the hot flush, a sudden feeling of warmth and perspiration followed by a sensation of chill. Hot flushes occur without warning at irregular intervals. Other physical symptoms include itching skin, constipation, heart palpitations, headache, dizziness, and insomnia.

For many women the most unpleasant symptoms of menopause are the emotional ones. Possibly because of a decline in their estrogen production, menopausal women tend to be irritable, anxious, excitable, tired, or easily depressed. Many are worried about what they see as a loss of femininity (although sex drive does not usually diminish). Some fear their husbands will lose interest in them, others look back with longing on the days when the house was full of noise and children. For others, fatigue is the expression of boredom and dissatisfaction with a life that seems to have lost its purpose.

Menopausal symptoms diminish with time and with acceptance of a new stage of life. Many doctors also administer estrogen to replace the hormones a woman is losing and help ease her physical symptoms.

Some doctors estimate that fatigue has an organic basis in one in every five patients who complains of it. If you suspect illness, make an appointment with the doctor at once. If he finds nothing wrong after thorough examination and laboratory tests, it is time to examine your emotional patterns and your life style.

BIBLIOGRAPHY

Beeson, Paul B., M.D., and McDermott, Walsh, M.D., eds. *Cecil-Loeb Textbook of Medicine*. Saunders, 1971.

"Chronic Fatigue," *Good Housekeeping*, Nov. 1970.

Fishbein, Morris, M.D., ed. *The Modern Family Health Guide*. Doubleday, 1967.

Galton, Lawrence. "Low Thyroid—Is It Sapping Your Energy?" *Family Circle*, Oct. 1973.

"Helping the Patient Who's 'Always Tired,'" *Patient Care*, Jan. 1967.

McGrath, Lee Parr. "How to Recharge Your Energy," *Family Circle*, Nov. 1972.

Sved, Dorothy, M.D. "The Surprising Facts About Mononucleosis," *Woman's Day*, Oct. 1973.

PART TWO

Emotional fatigue

As mental disorders continue to proliferate under the stresses of modern urban life, fatigue is increasingly identified with psychic and emotional causes. A potentially more dangerous, because less easily treated, symptom, psychological fatigue is the expression of inner tension, frustration, conflict.

It is also the result of a permanent or temporary inability to deal with life in a productive way. As mentioned, depressed people and bored people are particularly susceptible to fatigue.

For some people who are going through periods of great upset, feelings of tiredness may be a manifestation of what is variously termed battle fatigue, combat fatigue, or shell shock. Normally, these terms are used to describe the reaction of soldiers who have been exposed to sustained exertion and emotional tension. A soldier suffering combat fatigue is hypersensitive to noise, light, and movement, easily irritated, and does not sleep well. He is susceptible to headaches, backaches, gastrointestinal disturbances, depression, and withdrawal.

Obviously, not all soldiers develop combat fatigue, and a situation which is extremely distressing to one may leave another virtually unmoved. Investigators have found that factors influencing combat fatigue include emotional stability, prior ability to adjust, adequacy of training, level of morale, and degree of physical exhaustion.

The main cure for combat fatigue is to remove the source of the stress. Thus modern military leaders are careful to see that their troops are rotated at the front lines and that they are provided with enough rest, food, and sedation when needed.

In civilian life, combat fatigue is usually referred to as a "nervous breakdown" or "going to pieces," and it is generally treated in the same fashion: rest and sedation. Certainly there are few people for whom the stresses of life are so intense that they cannot continue to function. Yet it is important to understand the pathologic extreme in order to judge whether you yourself are headed in that direction.

Obviously, a situation of great stress such as a family illness is not a prerequisite for emotional fatigue. Yet it is possible that you are living under pressures that you are not aware of. Put your life under the microscope. Perhaps some daily situation which you consider not worth thinking about has gradually solidified into something large, and your fatigue is the tip of the iceberg.

9 THE TIRED HOUSEWIFE

The fatigue produced by the stresses of twentieth-century living is perhaps best exemplified by the "tired housewife," a creature who has been around for centuries yet who only now has been awarded a title of her own. Her particular kind of fatigue—often a combination of overwork, boredom, depression, erratic eating habits, and little exercise—causes physicians to throw up their hands in despair. Every week, women drag themselves to doctors' offices complaining of chronic fatigue. Yet the tired housewife is not even mentioned in most medical texts.

What kind of hope is there for the woman who must spend most of her waking hours chasing after children and pushing a vacuum cleaner around, yet still wants to be a sparkling dinner companion and responsive lover? Recently a group of physicians sat down together to compare notes and try to come up with some answers.

Profile of the tired housewife

"Tired housewife syndrome," they agreed, is essentially not a physical disorder, but an emotional one. The victim can be of any age, but most sufferers are in their mid-twenties and early thirties. The chief complaint: "I'm always tired, I don't know why, and I don't know what to do about it." An endless parade of other complaints frequently accompanies the primary one.

Although most women admit they don't know what is causing the fatigue, many are unwilling to accept a diagnosis of emotional upset. Some resent the suggestion that "there's something wrong in my head"; others simply feel better with tangible facts and logical explanations to cling to. Many women who feel unappreciated at home are looking for someone who will tell them, "You're working too hard, you need a rest."

Although every tired housewife has her own story, several patterns are typical:

• Jane is thirty-six years old, has three children and is a fastidious housekeeper. Every minute of the day is taken up with some productive effort, and frequently at night her husband will discover that she has slipped down to the laundry room to throw in a load of dirty clothes.

Jane's compulsive activity is not confined to the household. She holds offices in several local service organizations and is running for PTA president. One day a friend asks if she will take over driving the children to school for the week; Jane sits down in a kitchen chair and is suddenly overwhelmed by the realization that she is exhausted.

• Martha married her high school sweetheart, and at the age of nineteen found herself pregnant and unhappy. She never enjoyed babysitting, and her own sisters were much older. She does not enjoy taking care of her baby, nor does she like to clean house.

Her husband leaves the house at 8 A.M., tending to the baby first. Martha endlessly prolongs the moment when she must get out of bed. She dreams of the carefree days when she was going to football parties with Bill and taking off at a moment's notice for the beach.

• Joanne is almost fifty and has begun menopause. Friends tell her she is still attractive, but she won't believe it; after all, her husband is arriving on the last train from the city more and more frequently, and he hardly ever wants to make love.

While the children were home, they had something in common. Now, the reality she must face is that neither he nor they need her as much.

• Ruth was very happy raising her children, but always looked forward to the day when the last one would leave home and she could return to the career as a violinist which she interrupted to get married. Of course she could have been practicing and playing during those domestic years, but there were so many distractions, it was hard to find sixty minutes of solitude and a corner of the house where no one would be disturbed.

Somehow, however, she finds herself hesitating to pick up that violin. She's too old to become really good, she thinks, so what's the point? And the music-theory class she was going to take at the local university—wouldn't it be embarrassing to be a student among all those young kids? Now that she has been handed her freedom, Ruth doesn't know what to do with it.

• Anita is the well-groomed, articulate mother of two and a wife of a man on his way up the economic ladder. She has plenty of money for chic clothes, gourmet foods, expensive furniture, and private schools. But she longs for the days when she was arguing cases before the civil court judge—the only female member of the local bar association. She enjoyed holding her own in a man's world and is bored with her well-heeled but unstimulating existence.

How did she get that way?

Every tired housewife is tired for different reasons; the one characteristic they share is genuine physical fatigue, sometimes experienced from the moment they wake up. Superimposed on that fatigue are many possible layers of symptoms: anger, frustration, boredom, anxiety, depression.

Dr. Bernice Cohen Sachs, chief of mental health services, Group Health Co-operative of Puget Sound, Seattle, puts it this way: "I see the tired housewife syndrome at various ages and stages . . . the trapped twenties, the trying thirties, the fearful forties, the frantic fifties, and the sad sixties. There are reasons in each decade why women have difficulty coping with their roles, which may be manifested by psychogenic fatigue. I see the 4-F female: She's furious, frantic, futile, and frustrated."

Most of these women are not suffering severe psychiatric disorders, although the fatigue is usually rooted in emotional disturbance. Seldom will the capable doctor feel he must refer his patient to a psychiatrist; this will depend somewhat on where the patient lives, of course, on the prevailing attitudes toward psychotherapy, and on whether the patient can afford treatment.

It will also depend on how severely her ability to cope has been compromised. If she is merely having trouble facing the housework, she may need little more than a part-time cleaning woman. However, if life seems unlivable, she might do well to talk to a psychiatrist.

If poor relations with her husband appear to be the source of fatigue, a marriage counselor can often help both husband and wife gain insight into the situation—if they want to be helped, that is.

Other women gain strength and perspective from group sessions, particularly those launched by the women's liberation movement. Recognition that many other women are in the same boat is often comforting, although it will not do much to cure a genuine psychological problem.

What brings her to the doctor?

Few women will make a doctor's appointment simply because they are always tired, perhaps fearing a rebuke for magnifying what seems to be a minor problem. Most will bring up the matter in a casual way during treatment for something else—for example, on an annual trip to the gynecologist for a Pap smear.

"This patient often acts like the teen-age boy who comes in because he has wrenched his knee but uses the opportunity to ask me about what is really bothering him—his acne," says Dr. Joseph L. Bordenave, a family physician from Geneva, Illinois. "If the doctor is a good listener, eventually he will find out what the patient's true problem is."

Sometimes the tired housewife will try to be very offhand. On her way out the door she will turn around and remark: "By the way, Doctor, I meant to ask you. I'm so tired when I get up in the morning. Could you give me some pep pills or vitamins?"

Not infrequently, she thinks she is anemic or has a thyroid problem, but less than one patient in ten—male or female—is fatigued because of genuine physical illness. She may complain of headache, backache, weight loss, weight gain, stomach trouble, or insomnia. Some patients admit that they are depressed; others make a determined effort to give the opposite impression.

Often it takes a clever physician who knows his patient well to detect that she is suffering the tired housewife syndrome. No number of laboratory tests will reveal the problem, careful questioning and sensitivity to lightly dropped hints are far more productive.

The psychiatrist's viewpoint

Once a careful history establishes that the patient's trouble has emotional roots, there are two things to look for, explains Dr. Alfred Coodley, associate clinical professor of psychiatry at U.C.L.A. School of Medicine, Los Angeles. First, "What forces in the woman's life are impinging on her? Try to determine the cause of the stress that has led to her present clinical condition," he advises physicians.

Second, "What's her background? Ask about family and interpersonal relationships that existed when she was a child and an adolescent, and that exist now when she is a married woman."

If Dr. Coodley discovers from nonverbal clues that the patient is depressed, he will gently probe her state of mind, beginning with the question of whether she experiences particular mood problems. If she replies yes, he asks her how often she feels seriously depressed, and whether she ever feels that life is not worth living.

Suicidal thoughts usually lurk only in the farthest recesses of the mind of the tired housewife. Even so, Dr. Coodley urges the patient to be frank, and will ask whether she ever thought about committing suicide, and if so, how she planned to kill herself. Patients who have actually mapped out an elaborate suicide attempt are definitely in a dangerous situation. The more well organized and specific the plans, the greater the likelihood that they will actually be carried out someday. Naturally such a patient must be referred immediately for psychiatric help.

Yet the patient who plays with the idea of suicide is not necessarily a candidate for a mental institution. After all, who has not envisioned his own funeral? The tired housewife with anxieties, insecurities, and occasional thoughts of suicide may actually be using fatigue as a means of rationalizing why she cannot do what is expected of her.

Barbara, for example, had lived a reasonably happy fifteen years with her husband, when gradually they began to drift apart. They had raised three daughters together and had always presented the picture of the ideal happy family.

Of course everyone knew that Bob was the strong partner in the marriage—he made all the decisions, and he smoothed over the little irritations in her life as much as he could. Bob was a top manager for a packing corporation, and he was used to running a smooth operation, both at home and on the job.

Gradually, however, he began to drift away from his home environment. Transferred to another city, he found himself in the company of more stimulating people and more attractive women. The children were pretty grown and there was not the same pressure to get home at six for the family dinner. Eventually, talk of divorce hung in the air.

Barbara had always prided herself that she would never keep a man who didn't want her, so she agreed readily to a divorce. Bob moved into an apartment in the city and kept in close contact with the children, but came home only on weekends.

One day as he was about to set off on a business trip, he received a call from his oldest daughter. "Mother is acting funny, Dad. You'd better come home. She doesn't do the grocery shopping any more and she is too tired to fix dinner. She says she can't even leave the house, it's too much effort for her. All she does is sit around and crochet."

Barbara's fatigue obviously had nothing to do with lack of sleep. She had lost her ability to cope, having always depended on her husband for the heavy decisions. Eventually she was able to pull herself together, but not before long months of therapy with a psychiatrist who helped her work out her dependency situation.

Diagnosing the syndrome

Physicians agree that the way a woman responds to questioning is often more important than what she says. For example, she may claim that everything is fine, then start to get weepy at the mention of her youngest son, who has threatened to run away from home.

Dr. Leonard L. Lovshin, an internist at the renowned Cleveland

Clinic, gives the following counsel to this staff: "As you talk to the patient, watch carefully for sighing respirations, tics and twitches, inappropriate dress and grooming, and the habitual use of dark glasses when the sun isn't out. Examine how she looks and behaves in the waiting room, and what she does or says as she walks into your office."

The patient may enter the room slowly, painfully, and with great effort, suggesting someone who is overburdened or depressed. Or she may enter rapidly and aggressively, indicating a degree of anxiety or perhaps a competitive, hostile attitude.

"Also, notice whether she comes in with someone else—if it's her mother, she may well be involved in a dependency relationship. Look for the ease with which she takes her leave of the other person. There's always the possibility that she has come with someone else merely as a matter of convenience."

Does the patient sit down immediately on the edge of the chair in an anxious, expectant fashion, or does she wait for the doctor to ask her to have a seat? What does her face reflect? Is she flushed? Does she bite her lips, chain-smoke, or make restless movements with her hands or legs? If so, she is obviously experiencing some emotional conflict.

When a woman knows she is excessively tired all the time and presents the problem to her physician in no uncertain terms, there are various steps he should take in addition to searching through careful questioning for the source of the trouble.

Before writing off her fatigue as purely an emotional phenomenon, he should make a complete physical examination, including chest x-ray, blood counts and chemistry, urinalysis, Pap smear, and thyroid test. If the woman leaves the office with a clean bill of health, she will find herself much reassured by the knowledge that there is truly no organic basis for her complaint.

Of course, if the patient has been seeing the same doctor for years, all of these tests may not be necessary. Her physician may be alerted instead to search for conditions such as a viral infection which the patient is not aware of. A viral infection can produce the same symptoms as tired housewife syndrome for as long as eight weeks after the initial attack.

Certainly every doctor will not follow a standard procedure with each patient. And most will not administer a test simply because the patient asks for one, unless there is reason to suspect that something is amiss. Doctors are cost-conscious, too—or they should be. Certain tests are expensive.

For example, if a woman has recently had a baby, fatigue is hardly a matter for panic, and an extensive battery of tests will be a waste of time. A simple explanation of the physiological facts of life should suffice to make the patient understand that her body is reacting naturally to the trauma of pregnancy and birth.

Even when the doctor is sure that the patient has nothing physically wrong with her, he is making a grave mistake to dismiss her too quickly. After all, most people do not schedule visits to the doctor just to fill up a boring afternoon, and they like to feel that their problem, whatever it is, has been carefully considered.

A good physician will take the positive approach. Instead of saying, "There's nothing wrong with you," implying "Why are you taking up my valuable time?," he might point out, "I was successful in finding that there is nothing organically wrong. Obviously you are not feeling good, however, and this is a very real feeling. It's just that we must do a little more searching for the source of the problem."

Most patients are receptive to their doctor's opinion if it is presented in the proper spirit. The patient knows that she is exhausted and that she is not functioning well. If her doctor is frustrated by not being able to come up with a concrete explanation, and if this frustration is reflected in a "you're imagining things" attitude, she might do well to search elsewhere for help. Doctors are busy people, and not every one has the time, patience, or interest necessary to diagnose and treat something as elusive as fatigue.

On the other hand, the housewife should not expect the doctor to go through an elaborate workup just because she thinks her tiredness is a sign of cancer, for example. Most doctors know what they're doing, and if the patient really does have cancer, he doesn't have to perform hundreds of tests to find out. A patient should be able to trust her doctor's professionalism and intelligence, and not require a pile of lab reports to prove that he's right.

The doctor-patient relationship is a very fragile structure, and it is becoming increasingly so in this litigation-prone society. Most doctors will go out of their way to protect themselves against legal recrimination, and if anything, they will order more tests than necessary.

Some patients do not recognize that medicine is not an exact science; often there exists no definitive answer to a clinical problem, and the doctor is reduced to doing only the best he can in light of current knowledge. The patient who asks for miracles is being unrealistic, and may find herself wending her way through many physicians' offices before reaching the point of frustration.

Do you need drugs?

In this pill-oriented society, many people feel that whatever ails them should be amenable to treatment at the local drugstore. For the patient with tired housewife syndrome, however, this can be a dangerous course. Often the woman who asks for a tranquilizer or a stimulant is grasping for anything that will take away the symptoms of her problem and save her from staring into the bottom of a deep well.

It is only human, of course, not to want to confront what is painful. Still, it is unrealistic to think that a magic pill will eliminate all pain, and a wise physician will think very carefully before arming his patient with a prescription.

"I explain to the patient that it took a long time for her feelings to reach their present state and that no medication is going to make her feel better immediately," Dr. Sachs explains. "One has to be very careful about giving drugs to this type of patient, or to any other emotionally demanding patient."

Many physicians prescribe drugs, but only for patients who they feel sure understand the short-term benefits of medication. The patient must be one who comprehends that when she is feeling better, she will no longer need the drugs; their purpose is to help her over a temporary hurdle.

Understanding emotions

Many common expressions testify to our recognition of the relationship between mind and body. "My teacher makes me sick to my stomach" or "My uncle is a pain in the neck" are not taken literally; everybody knows what is meant. Most women are aware enough of psychology to understand that the emotions can surface in surprising ways. Still, many are unable to apply their wisdom to their own situation.

Alice was an active young mother of three who had an almost compulsive drive for accomplishment. Nothing made her feel better than cleaning the basement thoroughly or going through all her old clothes and sorting them out. She loved "getting to the bottom of things" and found it hard to go to bed leaving a job unfinished.

She had been raised in a strong church tradition, and "Look on the bright side" was the family motto. When a relative died of a long illness, it was always termed a "blessing" and a "relief." Whatever hardships came her family's way, they were prepared to look them square in the face and defy them.

One day Alice's five-year-old son was killed when a driver, backing his car out of a driveway, failed to notice him on his bicycle. Although Alice was shocked and devastated as any normal mother would be, she refused to "wallow in her grief," and even went so far as to have her bridge club over as usual the following week.

When she came to her doctor's office, complaining of constant fatigue, he was hardly surprised. Gently raising the matter of her dead son, he tried to make Alice see that she had tried to cut off natural feelings of grief too early, and that while she thought she was being brave and strong, in fact she was only hurting herself.

Eventually she was able to realize that she was much more shaken by the event than she would admit, and that she needed time to relax completely and recuperate. After a week at home with her parents, she began to face the pain that she had been camouflaging with fatigue.

Alice's case was a fairly straightforward one; basically she was an intelligent, sensitive, highly competent woman. Psychiatrists caution, however, that occasionally an emotionally disturbed person is better left alone. "Some people, whom we classify as conversion hysterics, derive certain benefits from their emotional distress," Dr. Lovshin points out. "These women cannot afford to be well: The cure would be worse than the disease."

Doctors often have to be good detectives to find out what is really bothering the patient with tired housewife syndrome, especially since she often doesn't have any idea herself. One Minnesota doctor's solution is to ask the patient, "What would happen if I gave you a $1,000 check and told you to do whatever you wanted for a week?" The answers he receives are often good indications of where the patient's troubles lie.

A woman who had recently moved with her husband from Florida to Minnesota replied eagerly that she would take the first plane for Jamaica and spend the week on the beach. This, along with other comments, indicated to the doctor that she was not adjusting well to the northern climate, despite her protests to the contrary. He phoned the woman's husband and suggested that they should take a brief vacation in the south as soon as possible. Eventually, he thought, his patient might learn to like Minnesota, but for the moment her lack of adjustment was the basis of her fatigue.

Another attractive woman of thirty-two said she would head for New York and spend all week window shopping, then finally buy herself a fur coat. Her doctor suspected that she longed for the days when she was single and earning money; he knew that she was very much tied to the household, however, and made a point of "always being on hand for the children."

When the doctor told her he thought she needed to get out more and suggested a friend who would be able to babysit two afternoons a week, she brightened up immediately. To her, as to many women, the doctor was an authority figure, and once he gave his consent, she felt released from guilt and responsibility.

Although chronic fatigue almost always has an emotional basis, often a simple change in household routine will go a long way toward relieving the problem. For instance, Janice had spent all ten of her housewife years following approximately the same schedule: up at seven, housework all morning, fix lunch for the kids, shop and do errands, fix dinner, relax in front of TV with Jack. Yet every morning of her life was agony: She hated getting up so early, was tired all morning, and finally came alive about 8 P.M., just in time to do nothing.

One day a knowledgeable friend suggested that she try shifting the pattern: get up at seven, but then go back to bed as soon as the family was gone, sleep for another hour or so, then get up and work. At night, when the kids are in bed and Jack is watching a ball game, polish the silverware, fold the laundry, or do whatever small chores are left from the morning. Janice had always considered it her duty to sit patiently with Jack, hands idle. When she took to doing small tasks in the evening, he raised no protest. Usually he was half asleep by that time anyway.

Certainly everyone must bend to the time schedules and routines established by society; although it might be fun to do the grocery shopping at midnight, most stores keep more conventional hours. An understanding of one's biological clock, however, can result in minor changes which make a major difference.

The money question

Nothing is more fatiguing than a chronic lack of money. With an empty pocketbook, the world is a dreary and burdensome place. Certainly many women who suffer tired housewife syndrome can lay their problem largely in the lap of poverty; they cannot make ends meet despite careful planning; an unforeseen expense has thrown the budget out of whack for several months; their husband is tight-fisted and refuses to believe how quickly the little expenses add up.

Nonetheless, some housewives are such pragmatists—by conversion or by nature—that they feel guilty about spending money on anything not labeled a necessity. If told they should try spending the night at a hotel in the mountains once or twice a month, they would protest that they couldn't afford such an extravagance with a perfectly good bed at home.

Many people have tunnel vision; they think that earning and saving money is what life is all about, and they look for their rewards in the wrong places. Although frequent short vacations may appear an extravagance, in terms of mental health they can be the greatest bargain in the world.

Everyone needs to be alone

Many women envision themselves as the central actor in a drama, without whom the play cannot go on. Although every human being needs privacy, a busy mother often finds it difficult to reserve a quiet moment for herself, and in any case would not risk being unavailable. Naturally, it is fatiguing to be on stage all the time.

"I always felt that if I retired to my bedroom and flopped out on the bed with a book, the household would go to pieces," a Seattle matron confesses. "The minute I got upstairs and shut the door, somebody would start whining somewhere. My son would be looking for his sweater and calling to me to find it, or my daughters would start an argument in the kitchen.

"One day I sat them all down and explained to them that mothers are not superhuman, they have needs like everybody else. I instituted a policy: For half an hour after dinner, no one was to disturb me, and any problems that couldn't wait to be solved should be taken to Dad.

"The children did not run to their father as quickly as they did to me—they knew better," she smiles. "Once I established the fact that I meant business, they left me alone. It's made quite a difference in my mental and physical state—that half hour of solitude gives me a chance to regroup my forces for battle."

The woman's next-door neighbor also complained of frequent fatigue, but her problem had other roots. Mrs. Friedman led what she considered a thankless existence; she held a full-time job in the local clothing store, and when she got home, ready to collapse from being on her feet all day, she had to fix dinner for a husband and three teen-agers. Since she made a point of not complaining, and in fact rather enjoyed playing the martyr, the family took her efforts for granted.

Naturally, Mrs. Friedman suffered chronic fatigue, though she would not complain of it directly to anyone but her physician. "When I told her how hard she was working and what a wonderful thing it was that she and her husband were sending their children to college, her face lit up like an angel's," the internist recalls. "It was only a little shot in the arm, this show of appreciation, but it did wonders for her."

The doctor realized that it would be uneconomical and impractical to have Mrs. Friedman come to his office every time her spirits needed a lift, but he was able to make her understand that her fatigue, while based in reality, was exaggerated by her unexpressed need for appreciation.

He took it upon himself to call Mr. Friedman, also a patient of his, and to tell him, "Your wife has got to have a little more feedback from the family. Otherwise she may collapse someday." Mr. Friedman, who dearly loved his wife, was rather startled; he worked very hard himself and never complained either. His first move, however, was to pick up the phone, call his wife at the department store, and announce that he was taking her out to dinner.

"Essentially, the patient must be helped to live with her situation or adjust to it," says Dr. Lovshin, the Cleveland internist. "Some of our best results are with women whose symptoms continue to some degree, but whose philosophical acceptance of those symptoms has been accomplished, at least in part."

Dr. Sachs of Seattle tries to "help change the woman's perspective so that she can cope." She gives her patients, who live under the shadow of beautiful Mount Rainier, the following example: "If you look at the mountain from Portland, it doesn't look the same as it does from Seattle, does it? Nothing happened to change the shape of the mountain; you merely changed your perspective. That's the same thing we are going to do with your problems."

Simplistic, perhaps, but sometimes the obvious way of looking at something is the last thing that occurs even to the intelligent person.

Getting out of the rut

Dr. Sachs maintains that the tired housewife syndrome has become endemic largely because of cultural patterns.

"The speed of social change in the past sixty years has far exceeded that of the preceding six hundred years, and women have felt these changes even more than men," Dr. Sachs points out. "In this society they play a multiplicity of roles. The modern woman is girl friend, mother, and homemaker; her husband's lover, housekeeper, companion, and friend. She's also part-time intellectual, woman of the world, community mover and shaker, property owner, and intermittent or partial careerist."

Obviously, men, too, play many roles other than breadwinner. Theoretically, a variety of demands should spell challenge, not fatigue. Yet a woman is more likely to feel that somehow her own identity has been submerged in all the roles she is obliged to play. She sees her education going to waste on diapers and dishes, she makes sacrifices for goals that she is not sure are merited. According to Dr. Aaron Beck, University of Pennsylvania psychiatrist, the result is "a sort of depletion depression brought about by an upset of the give-get balance."

Just as her children reach the age where they can be enjoyed as individuals, she finds them looking beyond the home for stimulation, Dr. Beck explains. This is the beginning of the "empty nest syndrome." A few years later her children do leave the house and the woman is totally unprepared for the loneliness and the inevitable depression which fills it like water fills a sponge.

The best solution to the situation, Dr. Beck feels, is not to let it develop in the first place. A woman should not wait till her children are grown up to develop outside interests but should start from the early days of her marriage. As the children grow older, she should spend an increasing amount of time away from them on things that interest her—doing volunteer work, taking classes at the local university, attending Women's Liberation groups, or whatever fulfills her own needs.

Although the tired housewife's problems are receiving a wider airing today than ever before, not all listeners are sympathetic. Dr. William A. Nolen, well-known author-surgeon, tells women that "most of you are tired for only one reason. You're bored. Your kids are in school and off your hands for several hours a day. You're not fascinated with the job of cooking two or three meals a day. Your husband is a nice guy, but after all, he has been around for a while. It seems as if all the challenge has gone out of your life, and you've nothing to look forward to but more years of the same."

For some or all of these reasons, he maintains, women demand a pill, a shot, or even an operation that will make them feel fifteen years younger. Unfortunately, however, "for the great majority of you there is no pill, shot, or operation that's going to help. Your 'tired-out' feeling has psychological, not physical, causes. No doctor can cure it; you have to do it yourself."

The important first step, Dr. Nolen suggests, is to break routine one way or another. Rather than spend money on iron, liver, or B_{12} shots, take the money and go out to lunch or to a movie, or both.

Apologizing for sounding harsh, Dr. Nolen admits that he, too, gets the "all-tired-out" feeling sometimes. "When I do, I first take a vitamin pill, which doesn't help, and then I take my wife and get away for an afternoon, which does."

Dr. Nolen is not alone in insisting that it is up to a woman herself to make the first move toward creating a more satisfying life style.

A first step is to get over the mental attitude that life is passing one by.

"Women think they're over the hill at any age—thirty, thirty-five, thirty-eight," comments Dr. Elmer Kramer, professor of obstetrics and gynecology at New York Hospital. "They think their youth is gone; they begin to see a few bulges here and there, perhaps see their husbands looking around. They've lost their initial drive and push."

Many women have unrealistic expectations of life and consequently react with frustration and unhappiness when they see that their lives have little in common with TV commercials or movie magazine stories. Disappointment is particularly a problem for women who reach the age of menopause and who fear the passing of their youth, their family life, their femininity.

When life becomes repetitive and mundane and a woman loses interest in the outer world because her own problems are too absorbing, she is headed for trouble. The unanimous advice offered by physicians whose ears are filled with these complaints: Do something stimulating. Dr. Nolen takes his wife to a movie, but for someone else, stimulation might mean joining the local bowling team or enrolling in a course in Egyptian art.

Many tired housewives have lived with their condition so long that they have forgotten what it's like to be stimulated. They can't even imagine what, if anything, might appeal to them. The answer for them is to deliberately pick something that sounds like it might be stimulating—even if only to somebody else—then force themselves to do it. They may well find themselves enjoying it. (Unfortunately, some women are so used to their fatigue that they are afraid to try change. They don't like being tired, but at least it's a familiar feeling.)

Many women find that volunteer work gets them out into the world and gives them a sense of involvement with something beyond their immediate needs. Others are happier with a paying job which offers tangible proof of their value and ability. One Cincinnati woman with considerable expertise in needlepoint finds that a part-time job at the local handicrafts shop has given her a welcome lift, even though she has to pay a babysitter for three hours each morning.

Children are not the only people who are entitled to having fun. Adults, mired in responsibility, may forget that they, too, have the right to play and to enjoy.

BIBLIOGRAPHY

Blackmon, Rosemary. "Fatigue, the Danger You Can't Ignore," *Vogue,* Mar. 15, 1972.

Nolen, William A., M.D. "When You're 'All Tired Out,'" *McCalls's,* June 1971.

"Pepping Up the Tired Housewife," *Patient Care,* Jan. 15, 1971.

Warshofsky, Fred. "How to Conquer the Blues," *Family Circle,* Oct. 1971.

10 SEXUAL FATIGUE: "TOO TIRED" IS NO EXCUSE

"Not tonight, dear, please, I'm too tired. . . ." A time-worn phrase which today is uttered perhaps equally often by both sexes. (Now that women are being told of their sexual rights, they are becoming less shy about asking what before they only silently wished for.)

The obvious first fact about sex and fatigue is that it takes more physical energy for a man to make love than for a woman. A woman can get by simply by not resisting her partner, while a man must reach an erection and maintain it.

In 1966, *Human Sexual Response,* by Dr. William H. Masters and Virginia E. Johnson (now Mrs. Masters)—the first major study of sexuality since the Kinsey Report—made news throughout the world. According to those two pioneers, both mental and physical fatigue can reduce a man's sexual tension to the point where intercourse is impossible. Mental fatigue, however, is undoubtedly the greater deterrent, during and beyond middle age.

"Reflected from the competitive male world, the loss of sexual interest paralleling 'the bad day at the office' initially results from mental exhaustion which only later may be translated into a physical counterpart," they point out. "As the male ages, anything with which he habitually is preoccupied necessitates the expenditure of significant mental energy and subsequently reduces his sexual responsiveness."

In older men, a personal, financial, occupational, or family crisis will usually repress severely any existent sexual interest, not just for the moment, but often for hours or even days. This sensitivity of male sexuality to mental fatigue is one of the greatest differences between young and old men. A twenty-year-old whose sexual interest is aroused is not easily discouraged.

"If the middle-aged male has the type of employment that requires essentially a physical effort, he long since has conditioned his body to these physical demands and there usually is relatively little involution in sexual activity that results from such occupational efforts," the authors comment.

Usually, if a man is too exhausted physically to make love, it is because he has been overexerting himself in sports, not in the office. Since most American men neglect to keep themselves in good physical condition, they arrive at middle age ill-equipped to withstand an exhausting weekend of violent activity, such as playing singles tennis in the hot sun. Frequently, the out-of-shape athlete will lose interest in sex completely for as long as two days after his athletic marathon.

Overindulgence in food and liquor, added to physical fatigue, can also make it unlikely that a man will want to make love. Under the influence of liquor, many a male of any age has failed for the first time to have an erection or to maintain one. In the middle-aged man, secondary impotence is frequently linked to excessive drinking.

Too much food can have an anesthetizing effect, and most people are not interested in making love on a full stomach. This repression of sexuality passes quickly, however, unless one is overeating constantly.

Vibrations of sexual disharmony

The old "I'm too tired tonight" excuse is only one of a number of ways in which people indicate that their sex lives are not in harmony, although it is one of the most common ways. Because the word *fatigue* is so vague and intangible, it often acts as an effective cover-up for deeper problems.

Unless one partner in the marriage is genuinely ill, sexual disharmony is a rare phenomenon in an otherwise mutually satisfying relationship. It does not exist in a vacuum; if a couple is having problems in bed, they are usually having other problems, too.

"While some may theorize in the style of which came first, the chicken or the egg, it is our firm conviction that marital discord precedes sexual disharmony far more frequently than the reverse," notes Dr. Barry R. Berkey, a Washington, D.C., psychiatrist. "Within the uncountable array of problems, those of a sexual nature not infrequently constitute the first recognizable symptom of what had already become a chronically covert discordant relationship."

Thus while "not tonight" may at first sound like a benign putoff, it can and often does spell a malignant marital problem.

Dr. Berkey lists five other categories of "fatigue factors" which are frequently enlisted as reasons for not wanting sex:

• "The pain ploy": Most popularly, headaches are used as an excuse for lack of interest in sex, although many variations are possible: "I think my back is acting up again."

• "Hazy and obscure": Here, a vague expression or comment is uttered so that the spouse hearing the remark feels bewildered and frustrated: "I feel edgy tonight; maybe tomorrow."

• "Chaste and shy": The unwilling partner exaggerates the possibility that friends, neighbors, or family may interrupt sex play: "The baby hasn't been feeling well, you know."

• "The altruist": One spouse protects the other's health by not having sexual relations: "I think I'm catching a cold."

• "Nature's way": From the wife, "I'm so sorry honey, but I just got my period." From the husband, "Darling, you know I have to get up at 6 A.M. and I've got to get some sleep."

Obviously, all of the above excuses are legitimate at one time or another. It is only when they form part of a repeating pattern that it becomes necessary to evaluate what is going on.

A number of physiologic and psychosomatic illnesses can produce fatigue. But Dr. Berkey points out that there is a big difference between people who "use" illness for extra mileage as a means of enforcing sexual distance and those who know that in a good relationship, illness need not prohibit sexual relations.

"The more solid the marriage relationship, the more stress the couple can endure secondary to organic or emotional disease without sexual disharmony resulting," he observes. "The less solid the relationship, the more rapidly fatigue will enter the picture as a symptom of sexual disharmony."

Fatigue can also be the honest result of overwork or of emotional stress, but even such situations, when prolonged, usually indicate that the marriage is in trouble. For example, a man who subconsciously wants to avoid coming home to his wife may work needlessly long hours simply to put off the final moment. A woman who no longer enjoys her husband sexually may insist on holding a job that she doesn't particularly like and that is not a pressing financial necessity.

The many masks of dissatisfaction

The man or woman who uses fatigue as an excuse to avoid sexual relations may actually be expressing any of several other problems. For example:

Boredom. After ten or fifteen years of marriage, a husband and wife can begin regarding each other as pieces of furniture, worn out and unexciting. Boredom with sex is the inevitable result of a routine approach in which neither partner tries to spark the enthusiasm of the other. Often apathy toward the home partner is reflected in a lack of interest in appearance, which can change dramatically should someone new come into the picture.

Hostility. Repressed hostility, often disguised as fatigue, may or may not be recognized as a symptom of marital strife. Hostility is usually regarded as a sinful or unacceptable emotion, Dr. Berkey points out; therefore many couples go to fatiguing lengths to deny it.

In fact, "Overt arguments are often avoided and delayed as long as possible, and a false cordiality is maintained until each spouse's denied anger can no longer be contained."

Fear. Pleas of fatigue to escape sexual intercourse may also express hidden fear of being taken advantage of emotionally. "Being open in lovemaking is to be trusting, and this involves—in the presence of a poor marriage relationship—a serious risk," Dr. Berkey remarks. "Trusting and then having one's trust betrayed by learning that one is only an object for the physical release of the erotic tension of one's spouse is a denigrating feeling."

When one spouse senses that the other is less involved in the love-making, he or she becomes fearful and begins to hold back. This fear of being hurt can and often does take on the mask of fatigue, according to Dr. Berkey.

Obesity. When fat people complain of being tired, they are expressing a physiological truth, but their reason for gaining weight in the first place may have been to avoid sex. Although most people who put on a lot of weight are not deliberately trying to repulse their mate, that is frequently the effect. The fat person is also relieved of guilt for not wanting to perform, because he or she knows that fatties are not in great sexual demand.

Other Reasons. Sometimes a woman will claim that she is too tired for sex, when the truth is that she knows she is at the fertile point of her cycle and is afraid of becoming pregnant. If she can't discuss the physiologic facts of life frankly with her partner, obviously their marriage leaves something to be desired.

Other women will claim fatigue on the grounds of "premenstrual tension" or because they have recently had a child. Obviously, not all such excuses are faked.

Men, on the other hand, will sometimes claim they are too tired to make love mainly because they are afraid they will not have a proper erection. This is particularly a problem in an age of sexual openness and at a time when women are demanding an equal share in sexual pleasure. If a man doesn't think he can satisfy the demands of his partner, implied or stated, he may plead fatigue rather than make a poor showing.

BIBLIOGRAPHY

Berkey, Barry R., M.D. "Too Tired for Sex: Fighting the Fatigue Factor in Sexual Disharmony," *Medical Aspects of Human Sexuality,* Sept. 1972.

Masters, William H., M.D., and Johnson, Virginia E., M.D. *Human Sexual Response,* Little, Brown, 1966.

I I THE AWESOME INFLUENCE OF STRESS

When a cave man found himself face to face with a threatening situation, he had two options—fight or flee. Unfortunately, the choice is not quite so simple for twentieth-century man. Frequently he is thrust into situations which don't allow for obvious courses of action.

For example, he hires a subordinate who turns out to be a pain in the neck, but who for the moment must be tolerated. Or he unknowingly moves in next door to a couple who stay up playing steel guitars half the night. Or he is forced to provide for a new baby when he has not received a raise in nearly two years.

Although there were no physiologists around during the cave man's day to measure his reaction to stress, we assume that he went through the same chemical sequence as modern man. For example, if a cave man noticed a wolf prowling around in the back yard, he would react immediately without thinking. Adrenal secretions would flash into his blood and bring strength in the form of both sugar and stored fats to his muscles and brain. On the spot, his full energy would be mobilized and his pulse, respiration, and blood pressure stimulated.

Muscles would tense, pupils dilate, skin vessels constrict. He would breathe more deeply, his heart would start pounding, and he would feel pressure on his bladder. In the end, he would either go after the wolf with a club, or he would retreat quickly into his cave.

Today we react in the same way, chemically. However, our options are not quite the same. The harassed apartment dweller, for example, cannot make a simple choice between protesting or moving. He is welcome to protest, but the landlord may turn a deaf ear to his pleas. He may consider moving, but may not be able to find the same kind of apartment for the same rent. Probably he will just sit tensely at home hoping that the neighbors themselves leave. And if he does that, he has to face the problems of adjusting his own need for peace to the racket next door, of putting a good face on things when he has company, of handling his feelings about how he deals with landlord, neighbors, and that company. And does he show anger to the noisy neighbors, or ignore the situation, or strive for some awkward compromise, or what? A simple annoyance can be fraught with such complexities.

Medical experts generally agree that a person who is chronically frustrated in his efforts to resolve stress is a good candidate for an early heart attack. If it's not his heart, he may register the stress by headaches, ulcers, asthma, ulcerative colitis—and certainly, chronic fatigue. Probably he will be a pill popper, possibly he will be temporarily impotent.

Some stress sufferers are able to work out their feelings in the bowling alley or on the golf course. Unfortunately, they then become more vulnerable to another common stress symptom, low back pain.

Why our civilization?

As medical historian Henry E. Sigerist points out, each century has had its own characteristic disease. In the Middle Ages it was leprosy and plague; syphilis took a terrible toll in terms of death and disfigurement during the Renaissance. The Baroque Era was characterized by deficiency diseases such as scurvy on the one hand, and by "luxury" diseases such as gout or dropsy on the other.

Tuberculosis and similar ailments marked the Romantic Period, "while the nineteenth century, with its tremendous industrialization, growth of the great cities and accelerated life tempo, spawned a wide-spread general nervousness as well as many specific neuroses."

Why has the phenomenon of stress mushroomed so quickly in a world where more people than ever are surrounded by comforts and conveniences? Dr. Aaron T. Beck, University of Pennsylvania psychiatrist, offers several observations:

"First, let me say that it's a world in which we are very conscious of things that produce stress: the competitive pressure on executives, the upsets caused by mobility, the difficulties of modern marriage, and so on. We also see evidence that many young people are less able or less willing than before to cope with adversities."

Stress is, nevertheless, an old problem, Dr. Beck points out, although today it is surfacing in more recognizable ways. Also, the term is now used in a sort of wastebasket sense to apply to virtually any emotional or mental problem after the event.

"For instance, if we have student unrest or an increased suicide rate, the phenomenon is first observed and then the cause is generally put under the term 'stress'—which can be as broad as economic instability or as highly specific as being rejected by a girl friend or boy friend," he comments.

Another reason which has been offered for the growing incidence of stress is that modern societies have largely lost the supports that helped people of earlier ages to endure physical and mental toil and hardship. In the words of writer Walter McQuade, these include "religious faith, sustaining frameworks of tradition and custom, a sense of place in the social order, a sense of worth derived from the exercise of craftsmanship, and awareness that toil, hardship, and suffering were likewise endured by the other members of the same community and the same social class."

Today, he points out, those intangible sources of consolation are virtually nonexistent in the lives of many people.

The lack of class distinction which is generally praised as a manifestation of our egalitarian philosophy has actually worked destructive effects in terms of an individual's sense of security. Despite the obvious disadvantages of social immobility, it is comforting to know that you belong to a certain class and that you have a rightful place in the world. Further, a system in which a man succeeds by what he does rather than by who he is has other disturbing consequences. A person who grows up with the idea that "any farm boy can become president" can create terrible pressure on himself. He is constantly wondering whether he shouldn't be striving harder to make it to the next socioeconomic plateau.

Although certainly rural societies have their pecking orders, the pressure is nowhere near as intense as in an urban environment where the communications media remind us constantly of what everybody else is doing and how well.

Investigations and research

The world's leading authority on the subject of stress, Dr. Hans Selye of Canada, has performed a number of interesting experiments in past decades. Dr. Selye defines stress as the nonspecific response of the body to any demand made on it.

His first breakthrough came with the observation that various kinds of insult to the bodies and nervous systems of laboratory animals had lasting effects in making them vulnerable to stress. The worse the stress, the stronger the reaction, in terms of adrenal overactivity, ulcers, shrinking thymus, spleen, and lymph nodes.

Dr. Selye's experiments with rats led him to believe that the endocrine glands, particularly the adrenals, were the body's prime reactors to stress. When the brain signals the attack of a stress situation, the adrenal and pituitary glands produce the hormones ACTH, cortisone, and cortisol, which stimulate protective body reactions. If the stress is a stab wound, the blood rushes irritants to seal it off; if the stress is a broken bone, swelling occurs around the break.

After the crisis, the body returns to normal. If the attack is prolonged, however, and if the defense system gradually wears down, deterioration, which Dr. Selye has christened the General Adaptation Syndrome, begins.

Why did nobody bother to study stress before Dr. Selye? His answer is that the phenomenon is so common that it never occurred to anyone to take a close look. Yet in addition to posing a health threat, he points out, stress can take years off a person's life by draining his capacity to withstand. Dr. Selye compares individual supplies of life energy to deep oil deposits; once the oil has been burned up for use in adaptation, it is gone forever.

Currently he is working with "anti-stress" hormones—catatoxic steroids—that produce enzymes which will destroy or neutralize toxic substances. The potential market for these substances, such as protection of industrial workers from dangerous fumes or mercury, is extremely broad, and many chemical manufacturers are backing Dr. Selye's efforts.

Research is also being carried out at the University of Michigan's Institute for Social Research, where one study revealed a considerable amount of occupational stress in the nation's industries. Of the workers surveyed, 35 per cent had complaints about job ambiguity; 48 per cent often found themselves trapped in conflict situations while at work; 45 per cent complained that they had too much to do.

Other occupational stresses included insecurity over having to do a task beyond normal scope; difficult bosses or subordinates; worry over responsibility for other people; feeling of nonparticipation in decisions affecting the job.

Personality types

For many years, researchers were interested only in the external factors implicated in the advance of heart disease—blood cholesterol, blood pressure, smoking habits, diet, obesity. In 1955, however, two California cardiologists, Drs. Meyer Friedman and Ray Rosenman, became aware that 90 per cent of their patients showed signs of inner tension. "An upholsterer came in to redo our waiting room, and pointed out that the only place the chairs were worn was at the front edge," Dr. Friedman observes.

When they began to put this finding to serious consideration, the cardiologists came to the conclusions that people can be divided into two major types, which they designate A and B.

Type A, the coronary-prone individual, is an intensely driving, competitive, restless, aggressive person who is used to getting things done. Type B is not necessarily passive, but he takes life easier, seldom loses his patience, and does not refer constantly to his watch. Although most people are a combination of Types A and B, usually one pattern or the other will predominate.

The extreme Type A is the kind who while waiting for the dentist will be making several business calls. He is filled with self-confidence and resolve and never ducks issues. He is seldom interested in money except as a token of the game, but the higher he scales the business ladder, the more he considers that his efforts are not sufficiently rewarded.

Type A's wife, who doesn't see much of him, is sure he is driving himself too hard, although he is very seldom sick. He is always on time for appointments; he is sometimes hard to get along with because his expectations of those under him are high.

He smokes cigarettes rather than pipes. He is not a reckless driver, but gets very irritated when the car ahead of him is dragging along. Type A spends little time just relaxing; when he indulges in exercise, it is usually a fast game of golf or a run around the park. He always returns from vacation on the day he says he'll be back.

Type B people are no less professionally competent than Type A's; in fact, they may reach the finish line first because they have a firmer grip on themselves and tend to make sounder decisions. Says Dr. Friedman: "A's have no respect for B's, but the smart B uses an A. The great salesmen are A's. The corporation presidents are usually B's."

Not surprisingly, perhaps, subsequent studies have shown that the Type A person is from two to three times more likely to develop coronary heart disease in middle age than the Type B. As Dr. Rosenman points out, "Type A is a sickness, although it is not yet recognized as such."

The two personality profiles worked out by Drs. Rosenman and Friedman are now widely accepted as reference points by the medical profession, although other researchers stress other factors in heart disease according to their own interests. Drs. Rosenman and Friedman do not yet have solid answers as to how one becomes either an A or a B, but they feel that both heredity and environment are involved.

Identifying stress

The Type A-B distinction is convenient from the physician's point of view, but other investigators have found another way of dividing personality types: the "sensitizers" and the "repressors."

In order to judge when such symptoms as fatigue, insomnia, heartburn, etc., are the barometers of stress, it is necessary to understand the difference between the two categories. A sensitizer is someone who is always attuned to signs of inner tension, and who is very much aware that his back hurts, his head aches, or his energy level is low. Repressors are relatively unaware that they are under stress, and may not find out till symptoms force them to pay a visit to the doctor.

Usually, stress is related to one of two previously existing situations: a sense of loss or the awareness of a threat. The first situation includes the obvious examples, such as death of a relative or loss of a job, as well as the drop in self-esteem that follows failure.

Threatening situations include anything pertaining to health, social status, personal situation, goals, sense of security. The husband who suspects his wife is running around will feel threatened, as will the professor who fears he will not get tenure, or the child who is afraid his parents will leave him at camp forever.

Although it might be supposed that stress triggered by external factors would be easier to identify and treat, Dr. Beck notes that some external situations develop slowly and are discernible only when a specific event brings them into the open.

For instance, he tells of a patient who was depressed because she felt her husband wasn't giving her as much affection as before, and who suspected he was seeing another woman. "I talked to the husband, and he denied this, saying he was giving her as much affection as always," the psychiatrist relates. "She continued to be depressed, and I wasn't able to get very far with her.

"Then one day she discovered that he had, indeed, been unfaithful to her for quite a period of time and that her perception had been correct. Once she established this and they had it out, she was able to cope with the problem, I was able to help her much more effectively, and within a few weeks she was over the depression."

The story also has a happy ending. After his wife brought matters to a crisis, the husband took stock of his situation and decided that his marriage meant more to him than his affair. He broke off relations with the girl friend, returned to the fold, and his wife never suffered another depressive episode.

Although this woman's reaction to stress was to become depressed, a number of people would react to the situation by becoming anxious. Depression and anxiety can alternate, and they can also coexist. However, the more severely depressed a person becomes, the more the anxiety symptoms recede into the background.

At the University of Washington in Seattle, psychiatrists led by Dr. Thomas H. Holmes have developed a "life-events scale" designed to measure psychological stress generated by various changes in life circumstances.

Their studies indicate that when a person scores higher than 300 in a single year, he may be headed for serious trouble. A total of 80 percent of those surveyed who exceded the 300 mark became seriously depressed, had heart attacks, or suffered other serious illnesses.*

Event	Scale of Impact
Death of spouse	100
Divorce	73
Marital separation	65
Jail term	63
Death of close family member	63
Personal injury or illness	53
Marriage	50
Fired at work	47
Marital reconciliation	45
Retirement	45
Change in health of family member	44
Pregnancy	40
Sex difficulties	39
Gain of new family member	39
Business readjustment	39
Change in financial state	38
Death of close friend	37
Change to different line of work	36
Change in number of arguments with spouse	35
Mortgage over $10,000	31

*"The Social Readjustment Rating Scale," below, was developed by Thomas H. Holmes, M.D., and Richard H. Rahe, and first appeared in the *Journal of Psychosomatic Research,* vol. 11, p. 216, in 1967.

It is reprinted with the permission of Microform International Marketing Corporation, exclusive copyright licensee of Pergamon Press Journal back files.

Event	Scale of Impact
Foreclosure of mortgage or loan	30
Change in responsibilities at work	29
Son or daughter leaving home	29
Trouble with in-laws	29
Outstanding personal achievement	28
Wife begins or stops work	26
Begin or end school	26
Change in living conditions	25
Revision of personal habits	24
Trouble with boss	23
Change in work hours or conditions	20
Change in residence	20
Change in schools	20
Change in recreation	19
Change in church activities	19
Change in social activities	18
Mortgage or loan less than $10,000	17
Change in sleeping habits	16
Change in number of family get-togethers	15
Change in eating habits	15
Vacation	13
Christmas	12
Minor violation of the law	11

Stress is good for you

In contrast to the physicians who are deeply concerned with the effects of stress on the nation's health, other researchers feel that stress has many beneficial side effects. Convincing evidence has been put forth that people under stress not only work harder, but are considerably more creative.

Writer Mae Rudolph, analyzing the situation in New York City, makes the point that "nobody loves bad air or traffic jams, but we flourish on what goes with them—and we will never know if New Yorkers could have accomplished as much or more if they had lived, Swiss-like, through several hundred years of tranquility."

New York University social psychologist David Glass, in the course of experiments on the effects of noise on efficiency, was amazed by "the discrepancy between repeated condemnations of the quality of life in the city and the fact that many people not only survive in these circumstances but actually thrive in and enjoy them."

The question becomes, then, whether a rich and creative life, inspired by the challenge of stress and nourished by steroid hormones and adrenalin, must inevitably demand a price in terms of our health. Dr. Hans Selye, the Canadian physiologist, offers the suggestion that stress is not necessarily detrimental, but that each person must gear his system to it through understanding.

Unlike Dr. Holmes, who thinks that change in itself is stressful even when it is for the good, two other researchers suggest that it is the quality of the change that makes the difference. Dr. Eugene Paykel of Yale University and Dr. E. H. Uhlenhut of the University of Chicago have ranked more than sixty different life events, divided into "entrances" and "exits."

Entrances include such new situations as the first months of marriage, a change of lovers, the birth of a child. Events such as death or divorce count as exits. According to these investigators, exits are more stressful than entrances, whether or not they make a less tangible change in life style.

Interestingly, rural people who live far from the noise and the crowds have just as high a rate of neurotic disturbance, and lower-income people are just as often afflicted by stress as wealthy suburbanites. The conclusion psychiatrists have drawn: The critical factors lie in a person's immediate situation—family, personal, or job—and seldom in environmental conditions.

Avoiding stress

Whichever rating scale seems more appropriate, the evident conclusion is that you should be aware of where the stress is in your life and try to adjust to it. In other words, if you are changing jobs, put off buying a new house. If you've just been fired, don't choose that time to experiment with marital separation.

And like the cave man, consider the alternative to fighting back, which is to flee. This is what Dr. Selye terms diversion: If the plane is delayed four hours, go home and take your wife out to dinner, then start again in the morning. If the date you've been looking forward to for a week cancels out, go buy the new record you've had your eye on. In other words, always consider an alternative rather than confronting the problem head-on.

As Dr. Selye points out, human beings are like automobile tires: They last longest when they wear evenly. People who notice that they have been keyed up for days on end should stop whatever it is they are doing and take a rest, even if it means deferring certain "musts."

The hormones produced during acute stress are meant to alarm the individual and gear him for peak accomplishments, Dr. Selye explains. Although they make a person alert for short periods, they cannot be used for recharging all day long.

In the end, it's the strain, not the stress, that makes for problems. Strain is the sum total of all the little stresses that a person didn't deal with too well or used up a lot of adrenalin in getting through: in other words, the "wear and tear" of life.

As Dr. Selye observes in *The Stress of Life,* "Man certainly does not get the feeling of happiness, of having completed his mission on earth, just by staying alive very long." The constant pursuit of comfort and security is "no adequate outlet for man's vital adaptation energy. Comfort and security make it easier for us to enjoy the great things in life, but they are not, in themselves, great and enjoyable aims."

Many people who are unable to cope with stressful situations find themselves overwhelmed with feelings of inescapable loneliness. This is especially true of adolescents and young adults, for whom there is no tomorrow, only the misery of today.

Psychiatrists have found that these unhappy souls usually learn to modify their reaction to stress simply by living through a few experiences. At first it seems that the loneliness will last forever, and that no one else in the world has ever experienced such a feeling. But once the lonely person gets through his first bout of unhappiness on his own, he learns that it is not such a unique and terrible thing. When the next episode hits him, he is better able to cope, knowing that he endured the same thing once before.

What happens to the career-oriented adult who finds himself the victim of self-engendered stress? "His trouble is an outgrowth of overemphasis on achievement and the notion that a person's self-worth is dependent on how much he achieves," Dr. Beck points out.

"In extreme cases, achieving becomes a life-or-death matter, and the individual is constantly generating anxiety, as if the ax were ready to fall at any moment."

If such a person can develop a more healthy attitude, learning from experience that achievement should represent only icing on the cake, then he is less likely to submit to the pressure of constant striving.

Not everybody is capable of introspection and self-analysis; however, most people can at least identify times when they need help. Aware of this, many business firms and industries employ industrial psychologists whose job is to lecture and counsel individual workers.

The common denominator in many cases of stress is loss of objectivity and perspective on life. Often merely talking to a psychiatrist, counselor, or minister allows a person to take a long-distance look at his situation, become less of a slave to inner drives, and develop ways of adjusting.

The technological approach

In recent years scientists have been involved in a concentrated search for new methods of fighting stress and its many manifestations—acne, high blood pressure, headache, peptic ulcer, and asthma, to name a few. Among the possibilities they have developed is a laboratory technique called biofeedback, which has shown promise in relieving not only stress, but certain medical disorders such as epilepsy.

The term *biofeedback* was coined in 1969 at the first meeting of a group that was promptly named the Biofeedback Research Society. People often apply the term in a grab-bag sense, because it actually refers to any technique using instrumentation that gives a person immediate and continuing signals on changes in a body function that he is not usually aware of, such as fluctuations in blood pressure, brain-wave activity, or muscle tension. The idea is that by watching how the disturbed body function is reflected on a laboratory instrument, the person can learn to control that function. Some examples of the biofeedback technique in action:

• An electrician with a dangerously arrhythmous heart lies on an examining table and learns to correct the beat by responding to a flashing red light;

• A Kansas housewife with a lifetime history of migraines learns to regulate the flow of blood in her head and hands;

• An insomniac musician learns to ease the tension in the muscles of his forehead by looking at the feedback signal produced by electromyogram.

All of this sounds like science fiction, and in truth, biofeedback is based on a startling new concept in physiology. Normally, we are able to control our skeletal muscles easily—your arm reaches out to turn on the oven, your toe kicks a pebble, your fingers turn the pages of the morning paper. Until recently, however, scientists were sure that man could not control his autonomic nervous system, that unseen regulator of interior processes such as pulse, glandular secretion, and oxygen consumption. It is through this pathway that the diseases of stress are often triggered.

Although some clinicians have been using biofeedback techniques for over twenty years, the subject first jumped into the public eye in 1968 with an article in *Psychology Today* on "Conscious Control of Brain Waves." This article described experiments by psychologist Joe Kamiya of San Francisco's Langley Porter Neuropsychiatric Institute in which subjects learned to turn the alpha rhythm of the brain on and off at will. Nobody could explain exactly how the phenomenon took place.

Shortly thereafter, Dr. Neal E. Miller, professor of physiological psychology at Rockefeller University, announced that he was able to train lab animals to control their autonomic nervous system through a system of rewards and punishments. His technique was first to drug the rats with curare to put their skeletal system out of action, then to use electric shocks as a teaching tool.

The rats, it turned out, could be taught to increase and decrease their heart rates, blood pressure, intestinal contractions, and other visceral functions. They could even send blood to one ear, making it blush, and not the other.

Dr. Miller maintained that his group's revolutionary experiments had "deep implications for theories of learning, for individual differences in automatic responses, for the cause and the cure of abnormal psychosomatic symptoms, and possibly also for the understanding of normal homeostasis."

His exuberant prediction was partly borne out by the experiences of other investigators who have applied the biofeedback technique in a number of interesting ways, with the help of modern electronics. For example, an ulcer sufferer swallows a tiny sensor which helps him control the flood of acid into his stomach. When the acid becomes excessive, he is warned by a meter sitting in front of him. Eventually, by concentrating on the signal, he may be able to control the flow of acid. Again, no one can yet explain just exactly how or why this happens. But the idea is that with enough practice, the subject can learn to apply permanently—without the visible signal —the technique he has mastered in the laboratory.

So far, most of the experimentation with biofeedback has been confined to the laboratory. Some advocates are hopeful, though, that the cost of the very expensive instrumentation might someday be reduced and clinics set up for treatment of the general population.

Autogenic feedback for headache

Of particular interest to many victims of stress and fatigue is the work on migraine headaches being done at the Menninger Foundation in Topeka, Kansas. Migraines are caused by dilation in the arteries of the head and scalp. After practicing for a few weeks, almost 80 per cent of headache sufferers using the biofeedback technique can learn to raise their hand temperatures by dilating the hand arteries. This prevents dilation of the arteries in the head and, consequently, prevents headache.

This form of "autogenic feedback" is now available at several places, including the University of Colorado Medical School, Chicago Medical School, Nova University in Fort Lauderdale, and Langley Porter Neuropsychiatric Institute in San Francisco.

The technique was discovered accidentally when a Menninger research subject was being trained to control her brain waves by electroencephalogram (EEG) feedback, reduce muscle tension by electromyography (EMG), and increase blood flow in her hands, as measured by hand temperature. The patient succeeded in raising her hand temperature 10° F. in two minutes, and she also recovered spontaneously from a migraine headache.

The hand-temperature trick is apparently easy to learn; one person who has had great success with it is Dr. Seymour Diamond of

Chicago, president of the American Association for the Study of Headache and the National Migraine Foundation.

The temperature training works best with young, well-motivated patients with true migraine, Dr. Diamond finds. "It's not much help to those with both migraine and depression headache—I prefer the term 'depression' or 'psychogenic headache' instead of 'tension headache'—and it seldom helps anyone over thirty. But I have about eighteen young patients who can actually abort their migraine headaches."

He has recorded even greater successes with EMG, a technique first used on tension-headache sufferers by Drs. Thomas Budzynski and Johann Stoyva of the University of Colorado. Electronic leads are placed on the forehead of the patient, who is lying on a bed wearing earphones. Any contraction of the frontalis muscle produces a tone in the earphones, and the higher the muscle tension, the higher the pitch. The patient's assignment is to keep the pitch as low as possible.

Although Dr. Diamond was originally suspicious of the work of the Colorado investigators, he is now an EMG enthusiast. "After buying EMG equipment, I started to work with certain patients in whom everything else had failed," he reports. "And about twenty intractable headache cases have responded remarkably. These are people who have been through the mill. They don't respond to anti-depressants, every other pharmacologic approach has been tried on them, and about half have had extensive psychotherapy as well, with no help."

The techniques used in tension control and migraine are also being used as an approach to chronic anxiety at the Langley Porter Neuropsychiatric Institute by Dr. Marjorie Raskin, who first became interested in this mode of treatment through her contact with harried medical students.

"Everyone can cope with a little anxiety, but the person who becomes afraid to do something because he thinks he can't control himself is the person I'm studying," she comments. "And that represents about 5 per cent of the population."

People suffering to this extent endure overwhelming fears of failure, to the point where they are practically afraid to stick their heads out the door. Headaches are frequent, insomnia almost inevitable.

"Chronic anxiety does not shorten your life. But people who have high intelligence quotients—and most anxiety victims do—don't live up to their potential," she observes. "Their ability to produce is killed."

The long-range approach

Tranquilizers are handed out almost as freely as aspirin to the stress-suffering population, but there is no evidence that they have any long-term effectiveness. The tranquilizer devotee may find that he feels better and is better able to cope when he is on pills; thus they cannot be denied a certain merit. Nevertheless, they will not help him work through long-range problems.

Many people will reach for the liquor cabinet when they feel under duress. Alcohol can certainly relieve tension for a little while; however, all too easily a person can launch a vicious cycle wherein the alcohol itself produces undesirable effects, such as depression or anxiety, and more liquor is needed to counteract these effects.

What about turning to family or friends for counsel? Dr. Beck points out that the problem here is that you can get either good or bad advice. "It would take a massive program of public education to train laymen to know what constitutes good advice," he comments. "An individual himself may know in a sense what good advice is, but he can't give it to himself. That's why psychiatrists go to other psychiatrists for help."

Not that everyone suffering the symptoms of stress needs to turn to a psychiatrist, he adds. "We do try to train our medical students to detect causes of anxiety or depression, and we also try to train family doctors to detect signs of stress in routine physical checkups or on office visits of patients for minor ailments."

What about minimizing stress for the next generation? The subject of child-raising is a constantly debated one, and the tides of opinion shift from generation to generation. At one time, children were considered miniature adults who should be treated as such. Then came the age of permissiveness and protection.

Many professionals now take the attitude that while a child needs love, he can also grow up straight and strong with a minimal daily amount. What he does need is the opportunity to confront various problems when he's young and to learn to cope with them.

"The parents, by intervening prematurely, may prevent the child from developing within himself the tolerance for problems or acquiring problem-solving mechanisms," Dr. Beck notes.

If a situation is too stressful, naturally the parents should intervene, but "the parent shouldn't do all the coping for the child. The idea is to create a learning experience so the child will be able to solve similar problems later on."

BIBLIOGRAPHY

"Biofeedback in Action," *Medical World News,* Mar. 9, 1973.

McQuade, Walter. "Doing Something About Stress," *Fortune,* May 1973.

————. "What Stress Can Do to You," *Fortune,* Jan. 1972.

Rudolph, Mae. "City Stress: Learning to Live in Condition Red," *New York Magazine,* Dec. 18, 1972.

Warshofsky, Fred. "How to Conquer the Blues," *Family Circle,* Oct. 1971.

"What to Do When You're Under Stress," *U.S. News & World Report,* Sept. 24, 1973.

I 2 HOW ANXIETIES WEAR YOU OUT

Nobody escapes occasional waves of anxiety, when for no apparent reason a vague, unpleasant sense that something is amiss or that something is about to go wrong washes over one. Anxiety often manifests itself physically as well—a heart that pounds, a hand that trembles, a palm that sweats. Psychiatrists think that these transient attacks are often caused by sexual fantasies which a person censors in himself, by fantasies of aggression or hostility, or by fear of loneliness.

But while normal anxiety is an unavoidable part of human psychological make-up, many people suffer anxiety reactions with a frequency and an intensity that are considered neurotic. According to psychiatrist Dr. H. P. Laughlin, anxiety reactions account for 12 to 15 per cent of the psychoneuroses seen in medical practice, and about one person in every four hundred suffers significant disability from anxiety reactions.

Dr. Laughlin divides anxiety reactions into three groups according to intensity. In an acute anxiety attack, often mistaken for a heart attack, the victim may go through a scene of dramatic panic, following which he actually loses consciousness. Such episodes typically occur without warning; suddenly the victim is overcome with extreme apprehension or fear, and he grows pale and begins to sweat. The event usually lasts no longer than an hour.

Between one and three persons in every hundred can expect to undergo an acute anxiety attack at least once in a lifetime, Dr. Laughlin estimates. Although many people live in fear of the next attack and may even avoid recreating the situation of the first one, generally these represent isolated instances in one's life.

A less severe form of anxiety reaction is the anxiety-tension state, where emotional and physical reactions are less intense and are precipitated by some kind of environmental stress. Soldiers at war may undergo a form of anxiety tension called combat fatigue, as discussed in the Introduction to Part 2. A singer on opening night may experience the same sensations, which can include unexplained fatigue, headache, or digestive upsets. Of course not all singers suffer acute stage fright, no more than all soldiers endure combat fatigue. People react in widely divergent ways to the same situations.

Although both anxiety attacks and anxiety-tension states are classified as mild psychiatric disturbances, many people who are mentally sound go through such episodes now and then. The point at which one can label a problem as neurotic certainly depends on how often such events occur and what prompts them.

Anxiety neurosis, the third category of anxiety reaction, is a chronic condition which is often accompanied by chronic medical problems such as indigestion or high blood pressure. "These can seem so dominant that the sufferer and the diagnostician may fail to recognize them as neurotic signs," Dr. Laughlin points out. "The neurotic person himself, often unwittingly, directs attention away from any underlying anxiety."

On the wide-ranging list of symptoms of anxiety neurosis, fatigue is one of the most common: It is very tiring to live constantly with ill-defined fears or tensions. The chronic anxiety sufferer is often irritable, tense, nervous, restless, a poor sleeper, and someone who often has trouble concentrating. Many are unable to perform sexually. Some neurotically anxious people eat too much, others find they have no appetite.

An anxiety neurosis is a problem which demands professional help. Frequently, the anxious person is not even aware that he has a problem worth identifying—he just assumes that everyone else goes around tense and fearful.

Sense of inadequacy

Frequently the rotten floor boards beneath feelings of anxiety rest on the unanswered question: "Am I good enough?" We are constantly measuring our attributes and achievements against those of others, taking inventories of ourselves. Few come out on top all the time and in every respect. Yet many people cannot live with this fact.

For example, a well-established and very attractive art director recently confessed that a few years ago, no matter how many people praised her looks, she was perpetually conscious that some women were more attractive.

"Sometimes I would go to a party knowing I looked like a million dollars—new dress, hairdo that satisfied me for once, good mood. Then I would see a woman who looked even more fabulous, to my eyes anyway, and I would search out the nearest empty corner and stare at the floor."

This lady, who was in her late thirties, was constantly afraid that men would inevitably be attracted to the younger women around. She also fretted over the possibility that someone brighter would rise up through company ranks and seize her job.

"Even if everything seemed to be going perfectly, I could have an anxiety fit over the possibility that things were bound to change for the worse sometime," she recalls with a laugh.

Everyone suffers attacks of self-doubt at one time or another, but when they become chronic events they are camouflaging a sense of unworthiness. Often this manifests itself in an inability to believe in other people.

"In the old days, if a man was supposed to pick me up at 8 P.M. and wasn't there by 8:15, I was convinced he was going to stand me up," the art director confesses. "When he did appear at 8:25, I'd chide myself for being so silly and for suffering all that needless anxiety. I guess it was just hard for me to have faith in the fact that a man could care enough not to stand me up."

Although frequently miserable, this woman was at least well aware of her insecurity, and eventually spent long and productive months with a psychiatrist. Other people are equally anxiety-ridden, only somehow they have managed to hook their fears onto something other than the real cause—a phenomenon which psychiatrists call displacement.

This is a phenomenon far from rare in unhappy marriages. For example, a young librarian named Anne who had recently moved with her husband from Houston to Chicago suddenly began finding fault with everything in her new surroundings. The weather was unbearably cold, the people weren't friendly, the stores were crowded, the streets were dirty.

Although Anne had always had the reputation of a complainer, in Chicago she began to outdo herself. Eventually, her coworkers were going out of their way to avoid her.

There may be plenty of things wrong with Chicago, but Anne's problems lay inside her. The constant fretting about external surroundings actually masked deep anxieties about a personal situation. Anne and her husband had been drifting apart for some time, but neither was willing to face up to the fact. Rather than clear the air between themselves and either get a divorce or build a new relationship, each developed different displacement techniques.

Many people who espouse almost any "cause" with unseemly enthusiasm are actually displacing personal anxieties. Sometimes the effects are at least partially beneficial; the woman who throws herself into charity work is presumably doing something helpful for an organization, is occupying her time in an unimpeachable way, and is receiving short-term relief from her anxieties. But the anxieties are still sitting there waiting to be paid attention to someday.

Fear of success

Several analysts of the women's movement have observed that anxiety in women is often rooted in a confusion of personal and societal expectations. In various ways, girls begin life with one toe over the starting line; they develop earlier, socially and emotionally, and they are better students than boys.

At the university level, however, the tide begins to turn. Most girls continue to perform well academically, but their hearts are already consecrated to the husband hunt, consciously or not. Among the graduate-school population, men heavily outnumber women, who by this time are either well on the way to the altar or are looking for some time-marking job in a big city.

This peculiar reversal is usually explained as a sign of woman's natural distaste for aggression, a distaste which makes her turn from competition. "All of our observations and predilections have traditionally supported the idea that women, in the long haul, simply do not have the constitution for normal competition; that, in women, the inner necessity to succeed which nourishes and sharpens the intelligence seems to be missing," notes Vivian Gornick, a leader of the women's movement.

"In all of the highly perceptive work done on the relation between motivation and achievement, none of the information contributed by women adds to our understanding of this powerful dynamic in human lives, because women seem unresponsive to the stimulus to achieve. In fact, they seem dominated by a profound wish to fail."

One woman who has devoted considerable attention to this phenomenon is Matina Horner, president of Radcliffe College and the youngest woman ever to hold that position. Several years ago Dr. Horner, then an experimental psychologist at the University of Michigan, began a study of the relation between motivation and achievement. She observed that while valuable information could be gleaned from tests given to men, results coming from female test subjects were irregular and disturbing. In particular, the women registered abnormally high on anxiety.

Some of her coworkers pointed to the data as evidence that "women are simply not capable of coping with achievement-motivation work," but Dr. Horner sensed that the problem was more complex. Women were not exhibiting a will to fail, she suspected, but rather an active, anxious desire to avoid success.

The desire to fail wells up from a deep psychological conviction that the consequences of failure will be satisfying, Dr. Horner explains. "These girls at Michigan were motivated by the opposite: They were positively anxiety-ridden over the prospect of success. They were not simply eager to fail and have done with it; they seemed to be in a state of anxious conflict over what would happen if they succeeded. It was almost as though this conflict was inhibiting their capacity for achievement."

Compelling evidence for Dr. Horner's theory has issued from other psychological tests. In a series of Thematic Apperception Tests administered at Michigan, each student was given either a picture to interpret or a story line to complete: for example, "After first-term finals, John (or Joan) finds himself (or herself) . . ."

From the answers emerged a vivid picture of the wide gulf between male and female concepts of success. Women usually associated achievement with loss of femininity, or with social rejection. Their responses suggested an attitude of withdrawal from challenge rather than a desire to respond. This fear struck the investigators as remarkable, considering that the young women were highly intelligent and came from homes where achievement was a positive value.

"Which makes great sense, when you think about it," Dr. Horner reflects. "After all, a girl who's not too bright and doesn't have much chance for success to begin with is hardly likely to be frightened by the prospect of success. Whereas, a bright girl from a middle-class home, knowing she actually has it within her possible grasp . . ."

The woman of the 1970s, if she is at all affected by the liberation movement (as who could not be?), is subject to a particular set of stresses being generated by the vibrations of new social forces. For those who are content with their pre-liberation roles, there is territory to defend. For those who are venting previously throttled frustrations and demanding change, there is the need to define the form that change should take.

In recent years the sanctity of the progression from love to marriage to children has been called sharply into question. Women are now called upon to make life choices that are meaningful in terms of the individual and not only in terms of social demands.

Yet women who have managed to arrange their lives in a personally satisfying fashion are still left with a sort of ideological hangover which is intensified by the ambivalent attitude with which many people continue to regard them.

Situational anxiety

While the chronic anxiety that arises from feelings of inadequacy can certainly be termed neurotic, situational anxiety is usually a normal though exaggerated response to change: new job, new wife, death of a parent, birth of a child. The anxiety disappears once the situation has stabilized.

For example, in the first few weeks after Frances moved to Italy with her new Italian husband, she found herself subject to frequent and unaccustomed bouts of tiredness, headache, and jitteriness. Although she would not have admitted the fact, she missed her friends and family at home. She was also frustrated at not being able to find work and distressed by the hostility she sensed on the part of her inlaws. All fair reasons for feeling tense and anxious.

Eventually these episodes began to diminish, and six months later, when she had found work and had won the affection of her husband's family, she reverted entirely to normal.

Another type of anxiety which has its roots in circumstance is the anxiety which afflicts many elderly people. Everyone knows the irritable and irritating old man whose complaining, querulous, angry attitude toward life drives everyone around him up the wall. He manages to keep the roots of his anxiety hidden from himself and from those around him. He tries to hide the resentment and anger he feels toward those he thinks are neglecting him, and toward himself for his weakness and failures.

Old age does not sit upon everyone with equal grace. Many older people are greatly disturbed by illness, loss of physical strength, and intellectual impairment. They have lost a sense of confidence in their own ability, and they find it increasingly difficult to cope with everyday problems. They may be poor financially. And beneath these layers of problems may lie psychological deficits dating back to childhood.

"In this context, the aged individual's disturbed and disturbing behavior—his 'anxiety'—is an elaboration of the 'emergency' emotions—fear and anger—brought into play in the search for aid," notes Dr. Alvin Goldfarb, geriatric psychiatrist at Mount Sinai Hospital in New York and chairman of the White House Task Force on Aging.

The older person who finds himself stumbling is frequently very much distressed by the need to seek help and protection, which he perceives as a loss of dignity, Dr. Goldfarb points out. Some feel guilty because they see themselves as burdens, while others become angry at a world that appears harsh and hostile. For many, the feeling that "I am old and no good" is expressed as "I hurt."

"They become suspicious of those who care for them . . . they may begin to exaggerate or exploit their ills and indulge in unwarranted complaining as a means of guaranteeing care or fending off desertion or neglect."

What help is there for these people? In addition to possible medical and financial assistance, they need somebody who can help them renew a sense of self-esteem and capability, Dr. Goldfarb stresses. "Any maneuver that encourages and reinforces the patient's conviction that he can handle problems, particularly problems of social relationships, fosters a sense of pride and dignity, assuages fear, and removes the stimuli that give rise to anger."

Although an understanding family can be very supportive, the mantle of responsibility falls most heavily on the patient's doctor, Dr. Goldfarb feels. Such an authority figure is in the best position to set up the psychotherapeutic relationship which these patients require. Unlike the traditional analyst-patient relationship, where a dependency is discouraged, it is often crucial in the rehabilitation of the older anxious patient, Dr. Goldfarb observes.

"In a sense, the security-seeking aged patient thrusts the role of parent upon the physician. To deny this role is to engage in a fruitless struggle that merely reinforces the patient's frustration and anger. Instead, the doctor should use this delegated authority in the patient's behalf."

Usually the only time requirement for this therapy is an extra fifteen minutes or so after the patient's regular doctor visit, as he is leaving the office.

Dr. Goldfarb's goals are twofold: first, to make the patient feel that the doctor's services have been won through the patient's own efforts, charm, wit, skill, or force of anger; second, to make the patient feel that he has won the doctor as an ally.

"Thus, patients leave the doctor's office with a triumphant feeling and the conviction that they have a strong protector," he explains. "They are strengthened, their fear decreases, their anger fades, they feel socially more acceptable, more self-respecting, more capable of productive behavior. From this point on, even small similar successes breed further self-confidence."

Older people frequently act as if life is a joyless and futile process and as if pleasure no longer meant anything to them. Typical comments: "Nothing matters any more . . . Nothing brings me pleasure and nothing brings me pain . . . I'd like to die and get it over with . . . I shouldn't need these medicines, they're just a crutch." Such comments are merely a disguised cry for help, a plea for care, sympathy, pity, and compassion. As Dr. Goldfarb points out, the façade of helplessness and hopelessness frequently masks a persistently hopeful sense of expectation. The complaining older person is appealing to those around him to respond to his needs, as he is no longer capable of changing his environment himself.

Drug treatment

Tranquilizers are carried out of the pharmacy as often as almost any other kind of medication. Yet despite the widespread use of these drugs, doctors are not agreed completely on what kind of person should be using them and who would be better off without.

"My first criterion for using an antianxiety agent is that tension is beginning to impair an important life area," Dr. James L. Claghorn, associate professor of psychiatry, University of Texas School of Medicine, Houston, reports. "If the patient complains of tension yet is functioning very well, his anxiety may be serving a useful purpose.

"Perhaps it is an indication of a life situation which calls for close scrutiny, such as marital or business problems. Evidently, the patient has sufficient strength to carry on; if you rush in with a medication, you may hamper your understanding of his life stress."

On the other hand, if the patient has really lost the ability to cope, the drug may calm him to the point where he can explore in detail the situation that is producing the anxiety, Dr. Claghorn points out.

Another psychiatrist, Dr. Donald F. Klein of the State University of New York, Stony Brook, feels that drugs are most warranted in the patient who suffers frequent and severe attacks of "anticipatory" anxiety. The latter refers to the distressed feeling that arises from anticipation of pain, whether of actual physical discomfort or of social humiliation or loss of self-esteem.

Anticipatory anxiety often arrives in the company of various other complaints, including fatigue, muscular tension, headache, back problems, heart palpitations, dry mouth, sweating, or gastrointestinal disturbances, Dr. Klein points out. "In terms of personality, many of these people find it hard to select a course of action and follow it through. They are chronically anxious and worried about what they are doing."

For the patient whose anxiety is an understandable response to a distressing life crisis, such as an impending divorce, and not symptomatic of a personality problem, a placebo is often as effective as a low-dose tranquilizer. One study showed that some 70 per cent of such patients will improve on either a drug or a placebo.

"Only when we treated chronic patients—with 'chronic' defined as symptomatic for six months or longer—did the placebo response drop and the drug response remain 65–70 per cent," observes the author of the study, Dr. Karl Rickels, director of psychopharmacology at Philadelphia General Hospital.

"In other words, the chronic patient benefits most from the anti-anxiety drugs. Moreover, in some patients with chronic mixed symptoms of anxiety and depression, we found some of the minor tranquilizers—in fact, even phenobarbital—to be helpful when the anxiety was very prominent."

Many patients are difficult to treat because it is not easy to distinguish cause from effect in the disturbing elements in their lives, the physicians admit. For example, Dr. Rickels tells of a forty-five-year-old woman who has suffered both anxiety and depression periodically for a number of years. The source of her distress apparently lies with her children, one of whom has a history of run-ins with the law and another of whom has a chronic disease. The mother is in good health, but takes Benadryl for hay fever.

"On the surface it looks like a chronic situation, but I'm not sure that drugs are the answer for this patient," Dr. Rickels observes. "Possibly she would benefit from a minor tranquilizer; however, in combination with the Benadryl, she might be left in an overly sedated state at night."

Certainly this type of patient should be closely observed, he notes. In time she may find that worries about her children are occupying a smaller place in her thoughts, and that she is functioning more effectively. On the other hand, the solution might be to refer her to a social-service caseworker and/or psychiatrist.

Valium and Librium are the antianxiety drugs most frequently prescribed, in dosages which should be tailored to the individual's reaction (in cases of neurotic anxiety, many physicians prescribe Equanil or Miltown). Some people's response to a tranquilizer is to become mildly confused, giddy, and irresponsibile, as if they had just put down two martinis. Other people are able to tolerate sedation with no apparent side effects.

One warning flag which all physicians should raise to the patient taking tranquilizers: Be careful about mixing them with sleeping pills, antihistamines, alcohol, or any agent which might intensify the sedative effect.

"I caution my patients about drinking, but I don't tell them they can't do it," Dr. Klein reports. "I tell them that getting drunk while taking the medication can be very dangerous, and that occasional fatalities have occurred that way."

Relaxing without pills

Certainly it is not necessary to rush off to a doctor or a psychiatrist every time anxiety attacks. For many people the antidote is to throw themselves into hard physical work, such as weeding the garden, cleaning out the cellar, or polishing the car.

What about other methods of coping? Psychologist Dr. Daniel H. Sugarman makes the following suggestions:

• Identify your feelings. Admit to the fact that you, like everyone else, are vulnerable to disappointment, anger, conflict, sadness. Say to yourself, "I feel hurt" or "I feel resentful." Recognition of the feeling can prevent it from turning into a mysterious ailment or into an attack against the people around you. Also, let other people know how you feel so that they don't blame themselves for your behavior. Expressing your feelings also relieves tension.

• Don't expect too much of yourself. The perfectionist is easy prey to depression, and his reaction to failure is to punish himself. Try to remember that perfection is not a normal human condition. Learn to live with an occasional unmade bed, an unfinished pile of correspondence, a sister who does not always approve, a husband who sometimes complains about dinner, a girl friend who doesn't like your ties.

• Postpone big decisions until you feel better and until you are calm and reasonable.

• Learn to help yourself out. People involved in work, hobbies, community or love relationships, who are moving with purpose toward certain goals are usually in better spirits than drifters. The crash may come later—after the wedding, after the move into the new house, after the promotion, when the sense of direction has been lost.

The way you follow up a triumph or a disaster often makes the difference between a return to a peaceful state of mind or a plunge into depression. Brace yourself for these periods of letdown and plan for ways to soften the blow. For example, when you get home from a fabulous three-week vacation at the seashore, clean out the basement, or start taking piano lessons. Do something that has a sense of purpose.

Self-help requires courage, dedication, and strength. Once you take the first steps, however, the rest follow much more easily. To avoid lapsing into self-pity, make a conscious effort to get yourself out of yourself. Go to a party even though you are tired; attend a community meeting even though you don't feel like talking to anybody.

To the above we might add a few more:

• Accept the fact that there are always people who are more intelligent, more attractive, more successful, richer, or whatever, and stop making comparisons. Instead, take stock of your own resources and capabilities and learn to value them. When feelings of insecurity send out vibrations of an incipient anxiety attack over a particular situation, say to yourself, "Yes, he's doing very well at the office and I'm having a bad day. However, I have lost forty pounds and look superb in my new three-piece suit, and he's developing a paunch." Eventually you may begin identifying with the winning side.

• Recognize that occasional anxiety is an inevitable part of life, and that even if you take up residence in an African jungle, far from the stresses of civilization, you will not escape it.

• While there is nothing wrong with temporary palliatives such as a stiff drink to take the edge off, consider ways of increasing your general sense of well-being for more permanent relief. These would include almost any sport, dancing, exercise classes, yoga.

Also think seriously about the many forms of therapy now available: traditional psychoanalysis, group therapy, women's consciousness-raising groups, biofeedback. Modern urban life is a rich breeding ground for feelings of isolation and loneliness, and no one should feel ashamed to seek help in dealing with emotional problems for which answers do not seem to be forthcoming.

• Instead of wondering why you're not getting anywhere, go out and do something. Look for volunteer work that will get you out of your own problems and into somebody else's. Day-care centers, for example, have a great need for women of warmth and patience who can help take care of the children of mothers who have to work. And male volunteers are always sought by the Police Athletic League, YMCA, and other organizations.

• Remember that anxiety is not always bad for you, and that it may signal psychological problems that need immediate attention. Also, anxiety can be the prelude to periods of growth. You feel tense when you crank yourself up to do something important or intimidating, but often you have the sensation afterwards of a pole vaulter who has just beaten his previous record.

It is also possible to control the physical manifestations of anxiety by learning to relax your muscles. Eventually you may even be able to drop off to sleep seconds after lying down.

Inner tension depends for its survival on the turn of a vicious circle, with many possible elements: fear, anxiety, overstimulation, frustration, sleeplessness, fatigue, talkativeness, anger, ulcers. Any one of these conditions produces muscle tension, which when disposed of will allow the other symptoms to disappear.

For example, next time you have insomnia, clench your fingers tightly, then loosen them very slowly. The more slowly you relax your fingers, the more deeply you will be conscious of the feeling of relaxation—and your control of it. If you train yourself to slowly relax the large, easily controlled muscles, eventually you will be able to control the smaller ones whose tensions are subtler.

There is no state of nervousness, worry, irritability, hate, aggression, impatience, self-pity, resentment, or jumpiness that is not dependent on tense muscles. While we can seldom turn off any of these unwelcome states by force of will, we can learn to relax them away by untensing the muscular tightness that supports them.

For example, how often do we toss restlessly in bed, unable to fall asleep because something is on our mind?

Very often when the brain is busily working overtime, its owner is reconstructing scenes or conversations of the day. In fact, he may actually be using his lips to form words. But if he relaxes his tongue, lips, and throat, it becomes impossible to think in words.

Likewise, if he is reconstructing a mental picture, he is using his eye muscles, even though his eyes are closed. By relaxing those muscles he will have a much harder time conjuring up the image. Or perhaps his thoughts are concentrated on a particular activity— his golf swing has gone to ruin, and he is mentally trying to correct it. Possibly his hands are actually tense as he grips an imaginary club. If he can relax those supporting muscles, he will be able to "turn off his mind."

Although the gradual-muscle-relaxation trick is guaranteed to succeed, patience is required; the technique cannot be learned in a day. Some of the work you won't even have to do yourself: each minute that the larger muscles are relaxed, more of the smaller ones will let go—even if you are not yet able to relax the small ones voluntarily.

Here are some suggestions for simple ways of relieving tension and promoting a continuing sense of "looseness." Try to follow them religiously for at least three weeks:

· Keep your hands and arms limp when not in use;

· Keep your face placid when not talking, especially your lips and brows, and don't use any more facial muscles than necessary when talking;

· Let your shoulders hang on their bones unless you are carrying something;

· Let go of any needless rigidity in your legs and feet when you aren't standing up or walking.

No matter what you do in the course of the day, you will do it better, with less fatigue and better judgment, if you hang loose. As you habitually relax needless tensions in your voluntary muscles, you will eventually feel the effects in the muscles beyond your control, such as those involved in stomach tension.

Every time you get into a tense situation, relax every muscle that you are aware of. After doing this a number of times, you will find it becoming almost second nature.

Changes of mood

Before leaving the subject of anxiety, it should be noted that, at times, symptoms indicate not difficult life situations or psychological pressures, but simple changes of mood. Everyone has his own internal clock; some people are edgy and fussy early in the morning, while others bound out of bed with a smile on their face. The biological clock has a strong effect on moods.

Thus a particular incident can evoke different reactions in the same person according to the time of day when it occurs. In other words, Mrs. Jones may find that at 10 A.M., the news that her son is flunking out of college is totally shattering. If he had only waited till 3 P.M. to call her, he might have received a more consoling reaction.

People's moods also fluctuate on a long-term basis, shifting back and forth from periods of relative contentment to relative depression. Most mood cycles run on a four-to-five-week basis, but they can run as short as two weeks or as long as several months.

In women, mood changes are often closely tied to the menstrual cycle. Many women find themselves anxious, irritable, and depressed in the few days before they start menstruating. In fact, a large proportion of crimes committed by women occur during the premenstrual period.

"I have seen many couples on the brink of separation, with the husband frustrated and utterly baffled by his wife's behavior," notes Dr. Sugarman. " 'Everything will be going smoothly,' is a typical complaint, 'and suddenly we're upside down and nothing I do or say is right.' Quite often, a pattern shows up in these discussions pointing to extreme premenstrual tension. Medication prescribed by a gynecologist usually relieves the disorder."

Our moods are controlled by certain enzymes in the brain tissue which scientists are now studying closely. When these body chemicals are not in balance, our moods change. In addition to biological factors, we are constantly reacting to our environment; for example, the sight of a park full of flowering trees on a bright April morning can gladden the heart, while the sight of children playing in the streets of a slum can be depressing.

Many working people drag themselves gloomily to the office on a

Monday morning, then their spirits rise gradually as the Friday afternoon liberation approaches. Other people who lead highly programed lives may find themselves blue on Sunday afternoon, when they have nothing better to do than enjoy themselves.

Seasons can also play on mood. The arrival of spring can be depressing to a person who is unhappy or lonely and who doesn't feel part of the earth's reawakening. The approach of the December holidays can work the same effects: For someone who is going through a sad time of life, the thought of Christmas or Hanukkah is not very cheering.

Bad weather is often singled out as the cause of low spirits, and in fact recent research at the University of Pennsylvania suggests that weather conditions, air pollution, and news headlines all affect mental health. In a survey of 879 Philadelphia area people, Dr. John H. Valentine and associates discovered that more people seek help for depression during periods of high barometric pressure, while more people get drunk on days of low pressure. Fewer homicides take place on sunny days.

Other scientists argue that weather is usually enlisted as a convenient explanation for moods arising from other causes. Certainly, if your best friend dies, no amount of sunshine will keep you from crying, while if you win the state lottery, a tropical downpour will not dampen your exuberance.

Impact of events

Obviously, the greatest mood changes are produced by events. Under the stress of overwork, shock, fatigue, or a sharp change in routine, people become hypersensitive, and molehills quickly turn into mountains. Often these overreactions lead to counterreactions, with explosive results.

"Much of the latter could be avoided if we'd make allowances during times of stress, but we often fail to recognize our emotional states," Dr. Sugarman counsels. "Sometimes, in fact, we are unaware of the loss or disappointment that sets off a depression."

Background, early training, physical make-up, current environment and activities all contribute to a person's moods. "Without the moods that provide life's coloring, life would be drab indeed," Dr. Sugarman points out. "Like colors, moods are neither good nor bad, right nor wrong—except as they work in context with the rest of the picture."

Unfortunately, he points out, many Americans equate cheerfulness with virtue, a broad grin with a "good personality," a happy frame of mind with the way things ought to be. But while the Declaration of Independence grants us the pursuit of happiness, it says nothing about where to find it.

"There are plenty of good reasons for feeling bad," Dr. Sugarman points out. "Anybody who is perpetually cheery has to be pretty insensitive to the way things are in the real world. In fact, feeling bad about the way things are is good—if it inspires us to work at making things better."

Many people make life hard for themselves by suffering needless guilt over mood changes. They think that unless they are cheerful every minute, something is wrong with them. Such people must learn that it is natural and human to feel low at times.

BIBLIOGRAPHY

Cronin, Mary, and Croft, Susan. "How to Live with Anxiety," *Cosmopolitan,* Apr. 1973.

Goldfarb, Alvin I., M.D. "Anxiety in the Aged," *Psychiatric Review,* McGraw-Hill, 1971.

Gornick, Vivian. "Why Women Fear Success," *New York Magazine,* Dec. 20/27, 1971.

Knight, Leavitt A., Jr. "How to Relax Without Pills," *Reader's Digest,* Feb. 1971.

Laughlin, H. P. "Psychoneuroses," *Encyclopaedia Britannica,* 1974.

"Office Therapy for Anxiety/Depression," *Patient Care,* Aug. 1, 1973.

Sugarman, Daniel H., Ph.D. "Are You Moody?" *Woman's Day,* Apr. 1972.

13 FATIGUE AS MASKED DEPRESSION

Every human being is depressed at one time or another, whether or not he advertises it to the world, but a growing number of Americans are "down in the dumps" so often it prevents them from leading a normal life.

Estimates vary, but at least 125,000 Americans are hospitalized for depressive symptoms each year, and another 200,000 are treated in doctors' offices or clinics. From four to eight million Americans are thought to be suffering depression of the kind that demands professional help for relief. When these people talk to a physician, fatigue is one symptom they complain of as often as any other.

Despite the awesome figures, depression is still not an "accepted" illness, as was proved dramatically in the case of Senator Thomas Eagleton, Democratic candidate for the vice presidency in 1972. The revelation that he had been treated for depression eventually brought about his withdrawal from the race.

According to Dr. William C. Ruffin, Jr., a Florida psychiatrist, depression and fatigue go hand in hand—particularly among the following types of patients:

• The adolescent whose short-term depression arises from his struggle for independence from family ties;

• The young adult who because of personality patterns is not getting enough satisfaction from starting a family or building a career;

• The forty to fifty-year-old whose visions of the future have begun to dim;

• The older person who finds it difficult to accept physical limitations on his activity.

Classifying depression

At what point does depression become a psychiatric disorder which demands medical attention rather than simply a transient phenomenon associated with the expected ups and downs of human existence?

Obviously, there are times when depression lasting for days or perhaps weeks is not only expected but normal. A young wife dies in a car accident, leaving a husband and two small children; a carefully nurtured business falls apart and the owner goes bankrupt; a desperately wanted baby is born with uncorrectible malformations. Who could not add examples to the list?

The line between what is usually termed clinical depression and ordinary reactive depression is often a tenuous one, and it is not always easy to pin the proper labels on people. Many physicians feel that determining the origins of depression is less important than recognizing and treating it.

"The doctor must ask: 'Is this depression understandable in terms of everyday life and experiences? Or is it so deep, out of all proportion to the event, that its severity can be recognized?'" says Dr. Zigmond M. Lebensohn, a psychiatrist at Georgetown University School of Medicine, Washington, D.C.

If the physician uses his common sense and experience, he probably won't even try to put the patient into a category, but instead will judge the degree of depression, Dr. Lebensohn maintains. Nevertheless, it is useful to classify the illness if possible, because patients with endogenous (internally generated) depression are the best candidates for drug therapy. Also, they are the most likely to make a suicide attempt.

"Clinically depressed" means not just blue, but virtually incapable of carrying out the routines of life. The sufferer may find washing his face and choosing a shirt and tie enormous chores. He may spend months brooding over the hopelessness of life, in the process cutting himself off from friends, family, and his usual forms of relaxation. Some people are clever at hiding depression from others, reserving their misery for solitude. Yet all the while they may be fighting back tears.

Recognizing the difficulty that even psychiatrists have in diagnosing depression, the American Psychiatric Association recently issued guidelines for distinguishing three types: neurotic, psychotic, and manic.

Neurotic depressives include a lot of people you probably know: people often considered of "weak character" by their friends and neighbors, who go to pieces as soon as problems begin to look insurmountable.

By contrast, a person who is psychotically depressed is often incapacitated not only mentally, but physically. Often such people suffer delusions or other thought disturbances. Their depression can be the result of internal derangements of body chemistry, or it can be triggered by external factors.

The third group—manic depressives—includes those people whose periods of depression alternate with spells when they are frantically cheerful, energetic, and generally on top of the world. Either phase may last for a period of days or months, and the two do not necessarily share equal time.

The majority of manic depressives swing regularly from high to low. Others stay high most of the time and only occasionally drop into gloom, and still others spend most of their time depressed. Many artists, both present and past, have been manic depressives whose creativity reached its peak in the manic phase.

Recognition of symptoms

A patient seldom appears on the doctor's doorstep with the sole pronouncement that "things haven't been going too well and I've been feeling low." Usually he comes in with any of a long list of other complaints, which can easily put the doctor off the trail of discovering the real illness.

Tragically, the patient who is allowed to drift along in a depressed state for months may end up a suicide statistic. Yet the risk of suicide is not nearly as grave as the suffering endured by a person who feels he is getting nothing out of life.

Certainly, fatigue heads most doctors' lists of symptoms which are a tipoff to depression. Many people suffer insomnia in addition to the fatigue, which is doubly frustrating; they are exhausted, yet they can't sleep. Other complaints include stomach cramps, loss of appetite, weight loss, headache, dyspepsia, constipation, dry mouth, anxiety, frequent mood changes, feelings of guilt or loneliness, and poor concentration. Numerous victims become socially withdrawn, agitated, more irritable than usual, inclined to excessive worry and pessimism.

Although a thorough physical examination will be taken as a starting point by a good physician, it will be of little help in ferreting out the real problem. Despite the battery of symptoms the patient may report—and may genuinely experience—there is no physical basis for his complaints. Of course, it is possible to be suffering a real physical illness in addition, which contributes to depression by reducing his general sense of well-being.

Not long ago a panel of expert psychiatrists and physicians spent a long day swapping experiences and trying to establish some guidelines for the average physician in the management of depression. Their comments show that depression walks into the doctor's office wearing a number of disguises:

• Fatigue is the number-one complaint "in all of the many ways in which patients tell you they are tired. If that complaint comes alone and without other symptoms, you are almost surely dealing with a depression of some sort. When other symptoms get tacked on, the most likely ones are gastrointestinal. After that are symptoms which are more a part of this patient's past experience and history. Virtually any symptom may be present, but most often one hears of a pain of some sort" . . . Dr. Robert Berkow, internist from Rochester, New York.

• "I have classified the symptoms of about eight hundred depressed patients over the last ten years. This summary indicates that disturbance in the form of either insomnia, difficulty in falling asleep, early awakening, or even hypersomnolence [excessive sleeping]. The most common symptom is early awakening" . . . Dr. Seymour Diamond, Chicago family practitioner.

• "What we're talking about might be loosely classified as the 'tired-blood syndrome.' It's the commonest thing I see in the medical clinic: people coming in saying they can't sleep well, or that in the morning they have a 'sick headache' or in the afternoon a 'little backache'" . . . Dr. Claude R. Nichols, Jr., psychiatrist from Dallas.

• "Depression is not a single syndrome. As far as we are aware, it's a number of syndromes. You might find a certain set of symptoms in a forty-five-year-old woman that would be quite different from those you would see in a twenty-six-year-old man" . . . Dr. Ronald Mintz, psychiatrist, Beverly Hills, California.

• Depression is frequently accompanied by an underfunction of one kind or another, usually by "loss or acute diminution of the four basic appetites: for food, for sleep, for sex, and for activity. All of these go down in patients who are depressed" . . . Dr. Philip Solomon, psychiatrist, Newton, Massachusetts.

Physical signs

Although fatigue remains the ⚡1 red flag warning of depression, Dr. Diamond's study of eight hundred depressed patients revealed that about 84 per cent complained of headaches which lasted all day but which were worse in the morning. He also found that nearly three in every four patients had lost from ten to fifteen pounds recently. Others had not lost weight, even though they had lost their appetite. They kept forcing themselves to eat in the hopes that it might make them feel better.

Of course there are always people—usually vastly overweight to begin with—whom no amount of crisis or tragedy can keep from the dinner table. When in a depressed state, they find that the only thing that gives them satisfaction is eating.

An indication of depression which is not generally known is dryness of the mouth or a bad taste in the mouth, usually reflecting a decrease in salivary secretion. Nausea and vomiting are other gastrointestinal disturbances which may signal depression.

Often a patient will reveal his mental state through a change in his physical condition. For example, the man with chronic ulcers will find that his ulcer is kicking up, although he has not altered his diet or his life style; the woman with a heart condition will suddenly start suffering chest pains.

It doesn't take an expert to point out that alcoholism and depression are long-standing acquaintances. Often it is hard to determine whether the alcohol is causing the depression or is a result of it. Many depressed people who have trouble falling asleep will turn to their liquor cabinet for help. This usually does little good, and the sufferer may become even more depressed while his alcohol consumption increases.

Sometimes the alcoholism will cease to be a problem when the depression has lifted; other times it may persist and become more evident after the depression has subsided. Also, bouts of alcoholism frequently coincide with bouts of depression—a person may go for months without touching a drop, then he becomes depressed and the liquor comes out of the cabinet.

"Agreed, some persons drink in an effort to drown out feelings of depression," Dr. Mintz points out. "But others who drink compulsively for other reasons may react to their inability to control their drinking with marked feelings of depression.

Dr. Solomon adds that in any event, a number of alcoholics are depressed as well as alcoholic. "If this is unrecognized, then you really can't help much in their alcoholism, and indeed you can do serious harm. To remove the alcoholism forcibly (as by Antabuse), without replacing it with psychotherapy or social aids, may throw some patients into suicide."

Occasionally someone will be taking a drug which acts as a depressant, although it is being used for other purposes. For instance, patients with high blood pressure may be taking one of several drugs—reserpine, hydralazine, guanethidine, methyldopa—that deplete the brain of essential chemicals and thus provide a biochemical basis for depression.

Corticosteroids such as Cortisone or ACTH can produce a variety of psychological disturbances, of which depressive reactions are but one type. Also, some physicians claim that oral contraceptives cause mood instability and depression in a few women. And the person who has been taking amphetamines, barbiturates, or narcotics and goes on the wagon almost always endures a period of depression as he withdraws from the drug.

Illnesses associated with depression

People suffering certain ailments will almost certainly be depressed, partly for organic reasons and partly because the thought of being very ill is depressing in itself. For example, hepatitis almost always goes hand in hand with depression during the long recovery period. So do most other disorders associated with persistent nausea. Even in cases of short-lived nausea, people frequently feel blue and discouraged.

Depression is also the companion of postcoronary conditions, cancer, or any incurable or chronic disease. And gynecologists are well aware that women are often depressed for several weeks after giving birth, during the menopause, and following gynecologic surgery.

The fact that many women are depressed after hysterectomy touches on the question of object loss, Dr. Nichols believes. A woman's attitude toward her uterus is closely bound to her concept of herself as a woman. For a man, on the other hand, the heart is very important in terms of self-image. A man who suffers a heart attack or a woman who undergoes gynecologic surgery has suffered an object loss, in the sense that a part of himself has been gravely injured or lost. It's like having a death in the family.

Depression following the loss of a loved one through death, separation, or rejection is easily understood, he continues. Object losses in terms of job loss and retirement also may put people in an agitated, depressed state. It's simple for the doctor to look at this the first thing: Who or what died and what is the loss?"

Every patient who is sick has lost something: first, his health, and second, the identity he had before he got sick, Dr. Berkow adds.

Not unsurprisingly, the more serious and prolonged the illness, the more likely it is for the patient to be depressed. Patients with cardiovascular disease are particularly susceptible. Doctors do not agree on whether the depression arises from the seriousness of the condition and uncertainty about the future, or whether there is a depressive personality type who is more likely to develop cardio-vascular disease.

The depression that accompanies organic illness is perhaps the only kind that can be prevented, when the physician gives the patient proper counsel and understanding. One study of patients undergoing "subtractive surgery"—loss of an arm, leg, uterus, breast, etc.—revealed that the incidence of depression was much lower in patients psychologically prepared for the loss. In most cases this preparation consisted only of a long talk with the surgeon prior to operation.

Many patients feel subconsciously that their operation is some kind of punishment or retribution for wrongdoing. If a father figure such as the surgeon speaks openly and kindly to them, they are much less likely to suffer depression after the procedure.

Likewise the patient who has suffered a heart attack: A sensitive and perceptive physician can help him to see that this period of withdrawal and apparent passivity can be put to good use if the patient is willing to reassess his goals in life and his investment in activities.

Easily overlooked

Despite the many subtle warnings visible to the well-trained eye, doctors admit that depression is one of the most difficult illnesses to diagnose. Particularly easy to miss is the patient who has come in over a long period of time with a variety of vague complaints with no organic basis. Another is the patient who responds quite well to treatment for whatever physical ailment he is suffering, then reappears in the doctor's office a few weeks later with a new set of complaints.

These people can mistakenly be taken for "crocks"—the doctor's term for patients who drift from office to office seeking treatment without really wanting to get better. Since their symptoms have no identifiable basis, the unpsychiatrically oriented or harried physician is easily tempted to scoff at their complaints.

"There is a general tendency in family practice to disregard the symptoms of these people," Dr. Diamond reports. "We tell ourselves that these people are not really sick and that it's more important to treat the acutely ill. Yet the depressed person probably needs our help at least as much as the others."

In identifying cases of masked depression, one of the major problems can be the patient's own attitude. Often he doesn't appear emotionally distressed, and may not acknowledge the fact upon questioning. On the other hand, he may complain of a symptom which doesn't seem to be enough in itself to justify a visit to the doctor's office.

For example, an eighty-two-year-old man came to a physician complaining of a cough that he said had bothered him for the past twenty years. The physician observed that the man was in superb health for his age, and that his medical history contained no record of respiratory disease or anything else that would explain a twenty-year cough. True, the man had a light cough, but he also had a slight cold.

Further probing disclosed that the man's wife had died recently and that he had been living with his son and his family. Now the son was being transferred to South America and the father didn't want to go. At the same time he didn't want to stay home alone. Most of his old friends were dead or living elsewhere, and he had nobody to talk to. Although he would not admit to depression, which he considered a "weakness," he was indeed depressed.

Physicians disagree on whether it is necessary to do a complete battery of psychological and laboratory tests on a patient who appears depressed, merely to rule out organic disease. Dr. Berkow thinks that the psychological tests widely used, such as the Zung depression scale, are of little practical value, and that the eye and ear of the physician are much more discerning instruments. He describes the typical depressed patient as follows:

"The patient looks grim or sad, his voice tends to be low, his speech may be slow and he demonstrates difficulty concentrating. Most important, he may choke up, change the subject to avoid weeping or may actually cry.

"He lacks enthusiasm and generally expresses an air of helplessness or hopelessness or self-deprecation. In other cases he may appear apathetic and unresponsive, may avoid looking at you or even turn his back. If the patient is agitated, he may be hyperkinetic [abnormally active], fidgety, fast talking (but disconnected), impatient and irritable."

Another looks for what he calls the "omega of melancholy"—the folding of the skin between the eyebrows in the shape of the Greek letter omega, which gives away the patient's state of mind.

What causes depression?

To date, this question has provoked three answers among researchers: Depression is an inevitable result of the pressures of modern living; it arises from inherent personality weakness; it is biologically determined.

One researcher believes that depression is a common phenomenon during a time of cultural transition and changing values, such as the past decade has been. Other researchers point to the increasing mobility of our society which makes difficult the formation of solid friendships.

Women are much more often the victims of depression than men —perhaps twice as often. Possibly women are more likely to admit that they are depressed, while men are more inclined to take refuge in alcohol. Also, our culture gives men more freedom to "let off steam" though anger and aggression.

Building on the theories of Freud and his early followers, modern investigators have been concentrating on a search for the psychological determinants of depression. Dr. Aaron Beck suggests that almost all thoughts of depressed patients are ruled by negative views of the world, of themselves, and of the future. Depressed people also tend to see minor obstacles as insurmountable hurdles.

A predisposition to a perpetually gloomy outlook develops during childhood, when a person first acquires attitudes about himself, Dr. Beck believes. People thus affected have sadly adopted the attitude that there is something basically wrong with them, and any time something happens to lower their self-esteem, they are propelled back on the road to depression. Something as simple as being reprimanded at work can bring on an attack.

For years experts have argued over whether mental illness has its roots in the function of the brain itself or in the interplay of outside forces. As far as depression is concerned, it now appears that a vital role is played by a group of chemical compounds called the biogenic amines, located in the brain.

Research has shown that depression can be a side effect of drugs that cause a reduction in levels of amines, in particular dopamine, norepinephrine, and serotonin. What trips off these changes is still unknown, although some researchers contend that it is an inborn defect of metabolism. Others feel that early-childhood experiences may themselves produce biochemical changes that lead to depression in adult life.

The role of heredity in manic depression is fairly well accepted, and the possibility that other types of depression as well may have a genetic basis—in other words, that the depression-prone person inherits his vulnerability from his parents—is now being considered.

Treatment

Two approaches are open to the treatment of depression: psychotherapy or physical therapy. Although the former is becoming available to more and more people these days, many doctors rely strictly on drugs, with a little counseling in addition. Others still favor electroconvulsive treatment for acute cases.

Whatever method is used, it is important for the patient to have a realistic estimate of what results can be expected and how quickly. Depression is not an unwelcome visitor who arrives one day and leaves the next; rather it is a condition which takes root and grows over a long period of time, and it takes time to get rid of it. As with almost any illness, there are cases of spontaneous remission. But in general, the patient should wait several weeks before deciding whether he is getting better or not.

Often the patient's second visit to the physician provides a good indication of how quickly he will respond to treatment. A young secretary under treatment with antidepressant drugs was discouraged at the lack of results after two weeks. On her second visit to the family doctor, she announced mournfully that she did not feel better and that obviously the medication was not working.

The doctor did not fail to notice, however, that his patient, who had come to him looking like a candidate for a woman's magazine makeover project, was now well attired and well groomed, as she had been in the past. In spite of what she said, the change for the better had already begun to take place.

Although for years psychotherapy and shock therapy were the only weapons for the treatment of depression, now a wide variety of drugs has been added to medicine's arsenal. Still, a recent study by the National Institute of Mental Health indicated that about 65 per cent of severely depressed people will be cured by no treatment at all. Although research monies are being poured into this field, scientific evidence and statistical proofs are few and far between.

Psychotherapy

Some doctors who feel comfortable with the psychiatric approach to illness and who are confident of their ability to deal with patients this way will undertake the psychotherapy of the depressed patient themselves. Others will refer him to a psychiatrist.

"What is really involved in psychotherapy—or 'the talking cure'—is the total person of the physician interacting with the patient, providing a feeling of sensitivity, of concern, and recommendations," Dr. Lebensohn remarks. "It may consist of education, explanation, assurance, and ventilation—letting the patient talk. This is where you start; then you go to the mild tranquilizers."

Formal psychotherapy has not proved very productive for acutely depressed patients. For one thing, it takes a while to establish the proper doctor-patient relationship, and if the patient is depressed to the point of being suicidal, he doesn't have time for this. Psychotherapy can be very effective, though, for the milder forms of depression related to specific neurotic problems.

Dr. Aaron T. Beck, a Philadelphia psychiatrist and leading depression researcher, finds that frequently the depressed person responds to simple tasks such as card sorting that help negate the feeling that "I'm a loser." Once the patient has mastered one task, he will be given something more complicated.

Dr. Beck also teaches patients to try and counter "negative automatic thoughts." For example, the patient who tells himself "I never do anything right" whenever he makes a small mistake is urged to put the brakes on this kind of thinking and instead to tell himself, "It's only human to make mistakes now and then."

Many depressed people have gone through one failure or ego-deflating experience after another, and have never learned that they are actually capable of fighting back. Two Alabama researchers will lead such people into an "antidepression room" and start hurling insults at them till they actually get mad. Anger is a good barometer of emotional condition; it indicates that the patient is no longer just beating himself but turning some of his hostility and aggression outside. (Freud's contention, still widely accepted, was that depression is hostility turned inwards.)

What can the family of the depressed patient do to help? Often a physician will confer with the family, explaining what they can expect and how they should treat the unhappy relative. Particularly with neurotically depressed people, the family can often help most by leaving them alone.

Many people make the mistake of being overly sympathetic. Relatives may try to minimize the patient's troubles by offering optimistic reassurance or "cheering him up" with special meals, little gifts, etc. Frequently this only increases feelings of guilt and hopelessness.

Electroconvulsive treatment

The mainstay of therapy for severe depression is electroconvulsive treatment, which will usually relieve depressive symptoms in four to eight sessions. Drug treatment can only mask symptoms.

Although in its early days ECT was a rather terrifying procedure, wherein a patient was held down so that he would not injure himself writhing with convulsions, today it is considerably less intimidating. First, the patient receives an injection of a mild anesthetic and muscle relaxant, which greatly reduces the convulsions. After electrodes are placed lightly over the ears, a split-second electric current is sent through the patient's brain.

Two or three minutes later the patient wakes up, completely relaxed, and walks away. The only side effects—and they disappear quickly—are loss of memory and mental confusion. Researchers are currently seeking means to avoid these effects.

Despite its record of successes, the use of ECT remains controversial mainly because we are still not quite sure how it works, or of its long-term effects on the brain. People react differently to treatment, too; one patient has trouble remembering her husband's name after one treatment, while another suffers no memory loss after five or six treatments.

Dr. Lebensohn believes that ECT should be used whenever depression continues for weeks or months without improvement, or when there is a sudden turn for the worse so that a person is totally incapable of coping with life. ECT suffers an undeservedly bad reputation, he maintains; it has saved countless lives, and when directed by a skilled therapist, there is no more dramatically effective treatment.

Dr. John Romano, founder of the department of psychiatry at the University of Rochester School of Medicine, agrees. He would use ECT for psychotic depressions under the following circumstances: when shock has been used before and has been effective; when there is a serious suicide risk; when there is danger because the patient cannot be under constant surveillance; when fast results are necessary for some particular reason; when the patient has suffered a toxic reaction to antidepressant drugs.

Drug treatment

Most sufferers from depression/fatigue are nowhere near the stage of having electrodes attached to their heads, however. By far the greatest number will be treated with antidepressant drugs, with or without psychotherapy.

Although almost twenty million prescriptions for antidepressant drugs were written in 1972, some clinicians insist that they are not being used as widely and effectively as they could be. The blame is laid chiefly on the shoulders of the family doctor, who is often unfamiliar with the many drugs at his disposal.

Other physicians maintain that drug treatment is overrated. Dr. Solomon makes the following criticisms: Many drugs take two to four weeks before becoming effective; some 20 to 30 per cent of patients will derive no benefit from the drugs and may even suffer side effects; drugs cure only symptoms and do not prevent recurrence of depression.

One internist who specializes in psychopharmacology admits that he uses placebos in the treatment of depression more than in any other illness, and that it's hard to tell the difference between the effects of the antidepressant drugs and the placebos. The reason, he says, is that mild depression has a tendency to remit spontaneously.

Antianxiety drugs can be helpful in cases where depression is mild to moderate, since often symptoms of depression and anxiety are mixed together. At the outset of treatment, many physicians will issue a mild tranquilizer (Librium, Valium, Equanil, Miltown) to help the patient get to sleep, along with a large dose of reassurance. Many cases of exogenous depression and even of depressive neurosis will clear considerably with such treatment.

Endogenous depression usually calls for the administration of a class of drugs called the tricyclics, or "mood elevators" (Elavil, Tofranil). These drugs work by increasing the effectiveness of brain norepinephrine.

If they are ineffective, the next step is a monoamine oxidase (MAO) inhibitor, whose primary action is the inhibition of the enzyme monoamine oxidase, but many physicians have strong reservations about the use of these powerful drugs.

Barbiturates are generally prescribed for the depressed person only with the greatest caution. Likewise amphetamines, although some physicians find small doses very helpful for depressed patients who have a great deal of trouble getting started in the morning. If taken after noon, however, the patient may have trouble getting to sleep.

A drug called Lithium has proved very successful in controlling the manic phase of manic depression. It has also been found helpful in staving off future episodes in patients who have already suffered an attack of depression. Because it can be highly dangerous if not properly administered, it is being used only in carefully selected cases.

One of the great dangers of drug therapy, of course, is that both patient and physician will let the drugs take over and will stop making efforts to uncover the roots of the depression. The patient is likely to say to himself, "I'm taking drugs now, they'll take care of my troubles," and the doctor may rely on drugs for some of the results that should be achieved through counseling.

One psychiatrist put it this way: "Now the doctor can get his nurse to give, say, B_{12} injections, or he can simply write a prescription for an antidepressant while he takes a trip to Europe."

Is depression ever cured?

The answer to this difficult question depends to a large extent on a person's concept of the cause of depression. Those who feel that it is essentially biologically determined maintain that even though individual episodes of depression will clear up, the dark cloud must inevitably return.

Most cases of mild depression are related to specific stress situations, however, and when the situation has been resolved, the depression will fade away. General practitioners estimate that some three out of four of the depressed patients they treat can expect a return to normal within six months.

BIBLIOGRAPHY

Cherry, Rona and Laurence. "Depression," *New York Times Magazine,* Nov. 25, 1973.

"Depression: Masked or Missed?" *Patient Care,* May 1968.

"Managing the Depressed Patient More Effectively," *Patient Care,* July 1968.

"The Pervasive Problem of Mental Depression," *Medical World News,* Apr. 20, 1973.

I4 FIGHTING BOREDOM

Next time you are conscious of an oppressive sense of fatigue, ask yourself: What have I been doing for the past hour? the past three hours? Is it the same thing I was doing yesterday? at the same time and in the same way? Will I be doing the same thing tomorrow?

Perhaps your tiredness is based not on overexertion, but on just plain boredom. Dr. Ralph R. Greenson, a psychiatrist, describes boredom as a combination of the following feelings: "A state of dissatisfaction and a disinclination to action; a state of longing and an inability to designate what is longed for; a sense of emptiness; a passive, expectant attitude with the hope that the external world will supply the satisfaction; a distorted sense of time in which time seems to stand still."

Boredom can result from two situations: an external world that is monotonous, and a frame of mind that reacts to a situation as if it were boring. In either case, individuals vary widely in their perceptions of boredom. A man on an assembly line may not find his work boring, because he refuses to let himself think about the fact that what he is doing is repetitious. Instead, he concentrates on the cold beer he will share with his friends after work. A wealthy socialite may find herself bored at a charity ball, while her young daughter is filled with enthusiasm and dances all night.

Occasional boredom is an inescapable part of the human condition, and people who claim they are never bored are rare. But many behavioral scientists feel that chronic boredom is largely a phenomenon of twentieth-century industrialized society. Our daily lives are full of examples of monotony: televisions and radios drone on for hours, half listened to. Superhighways stretch for miles with only a gas station or an overpass for diversion. Parking lots are monotonous, supermarkets all look the same, office and factory work can be very monotonous. Frequently, leisure time is monotonous, too.

On the other hand, the widely respected psychoanalyst Erich Fromm maintains that boredom is an internal as well as an external problem. Chronic boredom—"the illness of the age"—is a neurotic character trait, he says, which often seeks release in the form of drugs and violence.

First, let's examine what happens to a man when he is deprived of normal stimulation and is confined to circumstances which change little from day to day. When Rear Admiral Richard E. Byrd spent several months completely alone in the Antarctic, before the arrival of the other members of his historic expedition, he nearly went crazy.

"A man can isolate himself from habits and conveniences—deliberately as I have done; or accidentally, as a shipwrecked sailor might—and force his mind to forget," he wrote in *Alone,* the story of his adventure. "But the body is not so easily side-tracked. It keeps on remembering. Habit has set up in the core of the being a system of automatic physiochemical actions and reactions which insist upon replenishment.

"That is where the conflict arises. I don't think that a man can do without sounds and smells and voices and touch, any more than he can do without phosphorus and calcium. . . ."

Our knowledge of the effects of monotony derives largely from experiments in sensory deprivation. For example, during the 1957–

58 International Geophysical Year, the United States set up a number of scientific outposts in the Antarctic. Researchers on sensory deprivation studied the effects of the inhospitable climate—temperatures 100° below zero and winds up to 100 mph—on groups of scientists who agreed to isolate themselves for an entire year.

Most of the men spent every minute in the warmth of their quarters watching over the monitoring equipment. This lack of stimulation and change gave rise to many complaints; the men lamented the absence of physically demanding work and the lack of dangerous or challenging situations. Many found their memories beginning to slip; others were unable to concentrate or stay alert. Although they desperately wanted stimulation, many felt an increased desire for sleep. The end result of the situation: frustration and restlessness.

When the men got home, they were interviewed at length by a Navy physician, Capt. Charles S. Mullin, Jr. He reported in a psychiatric journal that probably "the lack of intellectual anergia [stimulation] and impaired alertness here bear some relationship to the factor of prolonged exposure to the 'sameness' . . . or, in short, the effect of the reduction in the amount and variety of meaningful sensory stimuli over a prolonged period of time."

Early studies

During World War II the Royal Air Force commissioned a study to find out why British radar operators on antisubmarine patrol sometimes failed to detect U-boats. N. H. Mackworth, who directed the study, discovered that these men usually spent hours on end keeping their eyes on a radar screen.

He set up a comparable laboratory situation in which volunteers were instructed to watch a pointer moving around a graduated dial and to press a button whenever the pointer made a double jump. Within a mere half hour, the subjects' efficiency had declined. The end result of the study: Tours of duty for the radar operators were shortened.

In this country, interest in the effects of monotony first arose after the Korean War, when it became possible to study men who had spent long months in prison camps being brainwashed by their captors. The lead was taken by two Canadian psychologists, Woodburn Heron and D. O. Hebb of McGill University in Montreal. They began systematically to examine the reactions of human beings to prolonged monotony, and in 1957 Dr. Heron made the first clinical report.

The subjects, male college students, were paid twenty dollars a day to lie on a comfortable bed in a lighted cubicle for as long as possible, with time out only for meals (eaten sitting on the edge of the bed) and for going to the bathroom.

These men wore translucent plastic visors which let in light but prevented pattern vision. Everyone was supplied with cotton gloves and cardboard cuffs worn over the arms to restrict perception by touch. Their hearing was limited by a U-shaped foam-rubber pillow at night, as well as by the continuous hum of an air conditioner.

Although most of the students had planned to consign their hours of isolation to academic projects such as organizing lectures or outlining term papers, they found themselves unable to think clearly about anything at all for any length of time.

When the investigators subjected them to a battery of mental activity tests, they found that, in almost every case, performance was impaired by the monotonous isolation. In addition, thought processes seemed to be affected; subjects became more inclined to believe in supernatural phenomena, for example. Some reported that they were afraid of seeing ghosts.

Like the prisoners of war who spent years in confinement in Vietnam, these student volunteers noticed that the content of their thoughts also underwent a gradual change. In the beginning they concentrated on the experiment, their academic work, personal problems, family and social relationships. After a while they began to reminisce about events in the past, making efforts to recall as much as possible. Many subjects resorted to counting numbers into the thousands to pass the time.

Eventually, some of the men reached the point where they were not thinking at all, but merely letting their minds drift into nothingness.

"Not surprisingly, the subjects became markedly irritable as time went on and often expressed their irritation," Dr. Heron reported. "Yet they also had spells when they were easily amused. In the interview afterward, many of the subjects expressed surprise that their feelings could have oscillated so much, and that they could have behaved in such a childish way."

After a long stretch in isolation, a number of volunteers began undergoing LSD-like hallucinations. At first they would see simple forms such as dots of light or lines, then the patterns would become more complex. One subject reported seeing "rows of little yellow men with black caps on and their mouths open." Eventually the hallucinations took the form of integrated scenes: a procession of squirrels with sacks over their shoulders; prehistoric animals; a procession of eyeglasses marching down the street.

Although in the beginning the hallucinations were a lot of fun and the men looked forward avidly to ensuing episodes, eventually the images took over to the point where it was difficult to fall asleep. Subjects also found that they would wake up at night and toss and turn in bed or get up and pace the floor. Many began talking to themselves, whistling, singing, or reciting poetry.

Fatigue and boredom

Since the publication of the Canadian study, many other investigators have explored the nature of sensory deprivation. One British study of railroad engineers is of particular interest in that it illustrates the tight relationship between monotony and fatigue.

Railroad engineers become weary on the job even though they are expending very little physical energy, J. Sharp Grant, author of the British Railways Board study, points out. Basically, the engineer's skills fall into two categories: "monitoring" and "tracking."

The engineer keeps one eye on a rapid stream of signals and the other on the needle of the speedometer. He has to be on the lookout for unexpected events such as the appearance of a herd of sheep crossing the tracks. In addition, he has to remember what to expect en route and which signals should be green at which places.

In the normal course of events, signals are green and railroad lines are clear, and the engineer has nothing to do but watch for the rare exception. This situation is perfectly designed for mental fatigue, which, as Dr. Grant points out, "arises not from overload of the human system, but from underload or monotony and boredom due to inaction, combined with stress."

How familiar we all are with this kind of stress-boredom fatigue.

A woman fidgets for hour after hour at the airport, awaiting the late arrival of a husband she hasn't seen for several weeks. A housewife stands in line at a supermarket, bored but anxious to reach the cash register. A librarian spends a dreary day rearranging the card file, a tedious job but one which must be done accurately and quickly.

Even interesting things become boring if overdone, as any urbanite who has spent restless days at the end of a long pastoral vacation can testify. At first the soul drinks in the quiet beauty of rural surroundings, but when day stretches out into endless day of sameness, one begins to long for the roar of traffic.

In the words of Christopher Burney, "Variety is not the spice but the very stuff of life." A British secret agent during World War II, Burney used self-discipline and mental gymnastics to endure imprisonment by the Germans.

"We need the constant ebb and flow of wavelets of sensation, thought, perception, action, and emotion, lapping on the shore of our consciousness; now here, now there, keeping even our isolation in the ocean of reality so that we neither encroach nor are encroached upon," he writes in *Solitary Confinement*.

When a person is exposed to a monotonous environment for a long time, his thinking is impaired, he becomes emotionally childish, his vision is disturbed, he suffers hallucinations, and his brain-wave pattern changes.

Studies of the brain indicate that normal function depends on a continuing arousal reaction generated in the midbrain, which in turn depends on constant sensory bombardment.

"It appears that, aside from their specific functions, sensory stimuli have the general function of maintaining this arousal, and they rapidly lose their power to do so if they are restricted to the monotonously repeated stimulation of an unchanging environment," Dr. Heron explains. "Under these circumstances the activity of the cortex may be impaired so that the brain behaves abnormally."

Exercise relieves boredom

People who make a point of exercising are well aware of the correlation between exercise and mental alertness or cortical tone.

Certainly, one way to perk up your brain and relieve boredom is to go out and take a brisk walk in the bracing air.

Sensations of movement play directly into the septal region, or pleasure system, of the brain. A psychotic person, for example, always has a malfunction in the mechanism that telegraphs sensations of touch and movement to the septal region.

In fact, according to Dr. Robert G. Heath, a psychiatrist at Tulane University Medical School, the apparent increase of boredom in modern life can be traced directly to our easy way of living.

"We don't get enough out-and-out tough physical exercise the way our forefathers did," he asserts. "We've become spectator sportsmen. I am thoroughly convinced that this contributes to our boredom, which I prefer to call 'anhedonia,' or 'lack of pleasure.'"

A few years ago psychiatrists working with the U. S. Bureau of Prisons developed personality tests which made it possible to spot "stimulus-prone" inmates: trouble-makers who were quickly bored and who needed continuous change. The psychiatrists found that when these inmates were assigned to varied, fast-moving work and recreation programs, trouble could often be avoided.

The role of aggression

In one of the most sensational murders of the century, a demonic young man named Charles Manson and his female followers brutally stabbed to death a pregnant actress and several of her friends in a self-proclaimed protest against the corruptions of the ruling class.

During the trial many people puzzled over the motives of the assailants, particularly of the three young women whose shaved heads and strident proclamations filled the pages of the daily papers. What could have driven them to such a sickening act of violence?

The startling explanation proposed by Dr. Erich Fromm: They were chronically bored. Dr. Fromm is one of several social analysts who have been trying to define the origins of aggression in human nature. He contends that the three most aggression-prone and neurotic character types are the sadistic, the necrophilic, and the bored. Boredom, he says, is the major source of aggression and destructiveness in twentieth-century America.

"Boredom, in this sense, is not due to external circumstances such as the absence of any stimulation, as in the experiments in sensory deprivation or in an isolation cell in prison," Dr. Fromm observes. "It is a subjective factor within the person, the inability to respond to things and people around him with real interest."

This type of person shares many characteristics with the person who is chronically depressed. Both feel powerless and resigned. They find little joy or happiness in personal relations, including sexual ones, and nothing in life or other people can spur their interest.

But while neurotically depressed people often anguish over feelings of guilt or sin, the chronically bored are apparently little concerned with their personal situation. They have little incentive to do anything positive with their daily lives. And while they can experience thrills, they are alien to feelings of content or joy.

Only a few people reach this extreme of boredom; most contract a milder form which can be compensated for by constant changes. "This seems to be the case with a large number of people in industrial society for whom the compulsive consumption of cars, sex, travel, liquor, or drugs has this compensatory function, provided that the stimuli either have a strong physiological effect, like liquor and drugs, or are constantly changing: new cars, new sexual partners, new places to travel to, etc.," Dr. Fromm points out.

For a fearful number of both rich and poor, there is only one way to compensate for boredom, and that is through aggression and violence, Dr. Fromm maintains. Violence provides immediate relief for those who have failed to develop normal human feelings of love and interest.

Other psychiatrists confirm that the boredom syndrome afflicts many teen-agers and young adults today, in varying degrees. Frequently, criminal behavior in these young people is the only outlet they can find for this boredom.

When the inhabitants of an institution for juvenile delinquents were interviewed, several who had taken part in stabbings or killings described their sensations as unique and exciting. The chief thrill lay in making somebody respond to them: a look of anguish, a groan of pain.

For example, in the Manson murders, Dr. Fromm suggests, "One of the main motivations for the stabbings was the sensation of making oneself feel alive in the act of killing, a feeling that was connected with sexual excitement for one of the girls."

Why is boredom an ever more noticeable phenomenon? Dr. Fromm theorizes that the structure and functioning of industrial society make it inevitable. Most manual work is boring because of its monotony and repetitiveness, while much white-collar work is too bureaucratic to satisfy the human needs for responsibility and initiative.

Worst of all, the "leisure" hours spent outside of the job are often just as boring as those which creep by during the working day. According to Dr. Fromm, leisure "follows by and large the consumption pattern, and is in fact managed by industry, which sells boredom compensating commodities. The difference is that boredom in work is usually conscious, while leisure boredom is unconscious."

Examples of leisure-time activities that can spell unmitigated boredom: a cocktail party; a ski weekend for someone with a tepid interest in sports; a singles cruise for someone who has been on too many of them.

Dr. Fromm feels that one way to reduce violence and drug consumption in our society is to make both work and play more interesting. However, this would require drastic changes in our social, economic, and moral structure.

"Man is a passionate being, in need of stimulation," the psychiatrist stresses. "He tolerates boredom and monotony badly, and if he cannot take a genuine interest in life, his boredom will force him to seek it in the perverted way of destruction and violence."

Individual initiative

Although the entire world may be covered with a blanket of monotony, some analysts of human behavior still feel that the burden of change rests on the individual. Dr. Henry Ward is a psychiatrist who bluntly informs his patients that "life is a simple case of being scared much of the time—or being bored."

Those who complain of chronic ennui are often as boring as they are bored, he points out. Frequently, people who whine that life is without interest have very limited interests of their own. They are afraid to step aside from their customary path; they are reluctant to expose their feelings, for fear of ridicule, rejection, or shame. So rather than brave the buffets of the world, they keep to themselves and to the territory they are familiar with.

But when life is easy and free of friction, it is not very much fun. Dr. Ward feels that children would be less bored if their parents would encourage them to make more adventurous choices in life.

"Take a children's coloring book where they fill in all the colors. That robs the child of an opportunity to draw his own pictures," he points out. "Like all of us, he chooses the easy way out. This way he doesn't have to risk anything. But he doesn't produce anything either."

What does Dr. Ward recommend to his patients who complain of chronic boredom? "I tell them to go to bed and not get up until they can think of something they really want to do. When they've done it, I tell them to go back to bed. They never take my advice, of course."

He also sends them to the library to look into a copy of Dante's *Divine Comedy,* where the fearful, bored petitioners at the gates of heaven are not allowed in, but are left to flounder in limbo, bored forever.

According to New York psychoanalyst Dr. Alexander R. Martin, boredom can often be traced to the early years, "where we find a reluctance to show natural feelings—crying, laughing, ebullience, enthusiasm—for fear of ridicule."

Eventually this state of affairs breeds a rather superficial, off-and-on kind of boredom characterized by an attitude of indifference, unconcern, and skepticism. People who develop this attitude resist motivation and will make no firm commitment to anything. Eventually, they may withdraw almost totally from life.

In the most serious form of boredom, the individual develops a hard exterior in order to protect his abnormally sensitive interior, and consequently loses feeling for everything, notes Dr. Martin, a former chairman of the committee on uses of leisure time of the American Psychiatric Association.

"I believe we have millions of people like this with us today. They are the tragically bored, jaded people. They miss the subtleties of life. They will travel miles to see the Cape Kennedy rockets, but overlook the firefly in their garden."

Not everyone is convinced that boredom is entirely a bad thing, however. In *The Conquest of Happiness,* Bertrand Russell maintains that in order to accomplish something worthwhile, a person must have the capacity to endure boredom and monotony. Modern man, he feels, is probably less bored than his ancestors, but more afraid of boredom and less willing to accept it as a part of life.

"Wars, pogroms, and persecutions have all been part of the flight from boredom; even quarrels with neighbors have been found better than nothing," he maintains. "Boredom is therefore a vital problem for the moralist, since at least half the sins of mankind are caused by fear of it."

All great lives and all great books contain vast stretches of monotonous territory, Russell claims. Therefore, he concludes, a quiet life style accords much more naturally with what can be expected.

"A life too full of excitement is an exhausting life, in which continually stronger stimuli are needed to give . . . pleasure. . . . A certain power of enduring boredom is therefore essential to a happy life, and is one of the things that ought to be taught to the young. . . . A happy life must be to a great extent a quiet life, for it is only in an atmosphere of quiet that true joy can live."

Boredom on the job

To find out if you are bored with your job, take the following test. It is based on a job-reaction study by a New Jersey management consulting firm, Roy Walters & Associates, specialists in job improvement.

	Yes	No
1. Do you avoid talking to your wife or friends about your job because you think they won't be interested?		
2. Do you find your job less interesting than when you first started?		
3. Do you have any qualms about the quality of the work you perform?		

	Yes	No
4. Do you occasionally lose interest in what you are doing while you are doing it?		
5. Do you often feel that you are marking time—just putting in time at your work?		
6. Is it hard to remember the last time that you looked forward to a day's work?		
7. Do you find it increasingly difficult to get to work on time?		
8. Do you find yourself taking a day off for no other reason than you don't feel like working?		
9. Does the thought occasionally occur to you that you would like to quit or change jobs because you don't like the work itself?		
10. Do you feel that your present assignment is a job in which nothing new can be learned?		
11. Do you dislike many parts of the work that you are actually doing?		
12. Do you feel that if you quit tomorrow your job would be filled easily and company operations continued unchanged?		
13. Do you find that you never think about your job when you are home?		
14. Do you think it difficult to rate how well you do your job?		
15. Do you feel a machine could do your job?		

	Yes	No
16. Do you feel your job is a dead end?		
17. Do you feel that you have little opportunity to suggest ways to make your job more efficient?		
18. Do you feel that when you do a good job on something, no one notices?		
19. Do you occasionally feel you are working harder to look busy than in accomplishing actual work?		
20. Are you confused about exactly what your job contributes to the over-all company product or service?		
21. At quitting time, do you find yourself more tired from the day's routine than from any work performed?		
22. Would you prefer to spend your time with people other than your co-workers?		
23. Do you often lose your place in what you're doing?		
24. Do you feel that an inexperienced person could handle your job as well as you can?		
25. When a suggestion is made about changing the way you do your job, do you first look for what is wrong with the suggestion?		
26. Do you worry that your children don't understand what you do and might go into the same line of work?		

	Yes	No
27. Does your job, as presently structured, give you reasonable opportunities for individual recognition?		
28. Do you feel that parts of your job could be eliminated without really affecting the work of your organization?		
29. Do you feel you have to have things checked unnecessarily by supervisors?		
30. Do you feel your present assignment is a job where you can continue to learn?		
31. Do you feel that you waste a good deal of time because of the way you have to do your job?		
32. Do you feel your work is checked too much?		
33. Do you get enough opportunity to correct your own errors in how you do things?		
34. Do you often feel that some parts of the job you do really do not make sense?		
35. Do you often feel that putting in extra effort is just looking for more problems?		

Of the 35 questions, if you answered "yes" to fewer than 10, you belong in that happy minority—Individuals who are not bored with their job, although he or she probably does not find it perfect.

From 11 to 20 "yeses" places you in the rather populous category of persons whose boredom with their work is a troublesome factor in their lives. Likely, these persons should consider attempting to make some changes in their method of work.

From 21 to 25 "yeses" denote a person highly bored with his job who finds large difficulties in reconciling his personal needs and his work.

Beyond 25, we have a tremendous mismatching of job and individual. This person's work bores him to sleep and it's difficult to understand how he stands it.

If you have taken the test and confirmed your suspicion that your job is a bore, you are probably wondering how you got yourself into such a position and what you can do to change it.

First, take courage from the fact that you are not alone. Job dissatisfaction surveys indicate that 60 to 80 per cent of workers are not satisfied with what they are doing and would gladly change jobs if they could. The reasons for this discontent are almost as numerous as the people holding the jobs.

"For some people, work is a sentence they serve each week to get the reward of their weekend freedom," notes Dr. Sol Warren, a psychologist at the New York State Office of Vocational Rehabilitation. "Such a man or woman has outside interests that are the motivational mainstay of his existence."

For example, Jose works in a supermarket twelve hours a day from 8 A.M. till 9 at night, with only a half-hour break for lunch and another half hour for dinner. He does this four days a week, during which time he barely sees his family and has time for nothing other than work.

Before he emigrated from South America, Jose was the owner of a dry-cleaning business. Not knowing English, he was forced to take a fairly menial job in this country—putting cans on shelves and keeping the store clean. Jose does not consider his job boring, since he doesn't think much about what he's doing. Instead, he concentrates on the three consecutive days off which he will spend with his family and when he will have time for fixing up the apartment they have just rented.

Jose's daughter also holds what many people would consider a dull job—she works in the typing pool of a large organization and spends most of the day typing address labels. She considers herself well paid, however, and is happy to have enough money to dress well and to save for a vacation. It doesn't occur to her to be bored. Also, she doesn't expect to be typing address labels forever.

For many people, boredom is the price they are willing to pay to get the things they want. They submit to almost any routine that is not totally unbearable. For others, a boring job poisons the rest of their lives.

"If the individual regards his job as a sentence to serve and has nothing enriching to look forward to after work is done, he will be unhappy and make others unhappy," Dr. Warren points out.

"The degree of the individual's alienation from his work depends on his philosophy of life. The time-server simply turns off his mind while he's on the job. The overqualified skilled worker or executive cannot do the same."

Jane is a key-punch operator who loathes her job. She would like to change professions but is worried that she might not be able to find a job at the same salary level.

Rather than try to make work as pleasant as possible—for instance by making friends among her coworkers—Jane keeps to herself and dashes off as soon as the clock strikes five.

She makes no effort to develop outside interests and spends most of her evenings watching television, hoping someone will call. Although an attractive girl, the bored, resigned expression which she usually wears repels most men.

In Jane's case the problem is essentially a personal one. In other cases it is clearly the job itself which is at the root of employee dissatisfaction.

Allen has climbed to the rank of corporate vice president in his paper-product manufacturing company and is very proud of the fact. Since his promotion, however, he has become distressingly aware that he has no real responsibility; he merely serves as a funnel for decisions made by his superiors.

Allen is starting to feel kicked upstairs, although he is quite happy with the salary, the fringe benefits, and the new office. Yet inside he feels hollow and lifeless, as if nothing he does really matters. His greatest sense of accomplishment one day was getting the copying machine to start up again without the aid of a repairman.

In Allen's case, the corporate bosses are at fault in not providing a competent worker with enough responsibility. Similarly, the auto-assembly lines provide classic examples of a loss of pride in workmanship that results from too fine a division of labor and a sapping of individual initiative.

What are the alternatives?

One possible escape from job boredom is to try a completely different line of work, even if it means taking a cut in income or moving to a less desirable location. The satisfaction derived from work that has real meaning for the individual might well make up for the other losses.

Certainly, there are many examples of men and women who have taken this kind of a bold step. The most famous case perhaps is the French artist Gauguin, who at the age of thirty-nine was working as a bank teller in France and who eventually spent most of his life in the South Seas painting.

Of course, it is easy for a young, childless couple to turn their backs on the materialistic world, head for the hills of Vermont, and open a delicatessen. They have much less to risk than an older couple who has raised a family and is heavily committed financially. Sometimes it is possible to fulfill only half a dream, yet half may be better than nothing.

For example, Robert, a forty-eight-year-old purchasing agent for an aircraft manufacturer, was distressed to find that work was becoming duller by the day. He knew his job thoroughly, but the company had recently begun cutting back on personnel, and he had little chance for advancement. His income was also very important to the family, as his wife did not want to work while their four children were still in school.

One day somebody asked Robert what kind of work he would rather be doing, and he didn't know what to answer. He had been a purchasing agent for so long that it seemed inevitable.

When the same person asked where he would like most to live, he unhesitatingly responded, "By the sea, where I was brought up and where we spend every vacation."

Eventually Robert put in a request for a transfer from the main office in Kansas City to a branch office on the Gulf Coast. He was still a purchasing agent, the squeeze at the top was even tighter, but he looked forward eagerly to evenings of strolling by the water and weekends of fishing.

Not everyone can pinpoint so quickly what it is they are missing. In the case of union members who issue long lists of sometimes niggling complaints, often the unrecognized plea is for recognition that the complainer is a man and not a machine.

Run-of-the-mill office complaints often reflect the same need for recognition and responsibility, notes Lee A. Parent, director of personnel and office services of the American Medical Association. For example, a secretary may find that nothing is right about her new typewriter. Or she may protest that there is too much noise in the office, or that her supervisor doesn't like her.

"Of course, individuals differ. Many employees are passive and only want to do what they are told to do," Mr. Parent points out. "Others are ambitious and will tend to do their jobs in their own way. It is important to take the difference between the passive and aggressive type of employee into account when evaluating and working to alleviate job boredom."

Mr. Parent's suggestion: An employee should never be assigned a job responsibility until he and the supervisor have sat down and discussed it. "The supervisor listens to the employee's ideas of how the objective can best be accomplished. When I'm the supervisor, the employee may end up doing it my way, but I will have considered his way. It takes longer but it results in a better quality of work."

Another suggestion: Modify jobs by delegating special responsibilities besides those regularly assigned. If the girl who makes the coffee every day starts to act bored and dissatisfied at coffee-making time, put her in charge of buying the coffee and give her time once a week to go and make the purchases.

Traditionally, employers have not been particularly concerned about personnel motivation. They figured that a pay check was all the satisfaction anybody needed.

Now, however, they have begun to turn an ear toward the behavioral psychologists, who admonish that work without personal involvement breeds apathy. In twentieth-century America, most workers do not have to worry about the primitive needs for food, shelter, and security. The satisfactions they seek represent a higher level of need.

According to a Yale scientist who has studied job motivation, Dr. Chris Argysis, "The employee must be provided more 'power' over his own work environment. Therefore he must be given responsibility, authority, and increased control over the decision-making that affects his immediate work environment. He must become self-responsible."

BIBLIOGRAPHY

Chew, Peter T. "Ten Ways You Can Cheat Boredom," *Science Digest*, Dec. 1972.

Churchill, Judith Chase. "How to Do More Work With Less Fatigue," *Woman's Home Companion*, Jan. 1953.

Fromm, Erich. "The Erich Fromm Theory of Aggression," *New York Times Magazine*, Feb. 27, 1972.

Grant, J. Sharp. "Concepts of Fatigue and Vigilance in Relation to Railway Operation," *Ergonomics*, 1971, vol. 14, no. 1.

Heron, Woodburn. "The Pathology of Boredom," *Scientific American*, Jan. 1957.

McGrath, Lee Parr. "How to Recharge Your Energy," *Family Circle*, Nov. 1972.

McKenna, Ken. "If Creeping Boredom Is Your Work Problem . . ." *Today's Health*, Aug. 1972.

I5 CONCLUSION

Chronic fatigue can be cured only by understanding and attacking its deep-rooted causes, but various emergency measures can give you the quick energy boost you need to get through a morning of meetings or a long evening at the opera:

- Lie down with your feet up for ten minutes, eyes closed.
- Take a cold shower. If you are tense as well as tired, take a hot bath first, then a cold shower.
- Walk quickly or run around the block, taking deep breaths of air. Or just open the window and breathe deeply.
- Start thinking about a pleasant event scheduled for the future—a dinner party, a wedding, a trip.
- Break your daily eating patterns—have pizza for lunch instead of cottage cheese.
- Call an old friend you've been meaning to talk to for a long time.
- Get the chores you dislike out of the way early in the day.

Although these simple measures can provide the necessary jolt, essentially they represent only patches on the threadbare tire. Let's take a look at the real problems and how to deal with them on a long-range basis. An understanding of fatigue demands careful self-appraisal, analysis of what the day consists of, and which demands or habits may be causing undue wear and tear.

Fatigue, as experts have discovered, is not the inevitable consequence of a certain amount of energy expenditure, but rather reflects a person's assessment of his own situation. If he is doing a job for which he feels poorly qualified or doesn't enjoy, he will find it tiring, no matter how little physical effort is involved.

Knowledge of this fact should be applied directly to the way in which time is budgeted. Our bodies are controlled by a circadian rhythm which is synchronized with the turn of the earth, but which is set slightly differently for each person. Possibly you are trying to force your schedule into a pattern that is unnatural for you, and you would really be happier washing windows at 6 A.M. and going to bed at 9 P.M. Perhaps the solution is to take a short nap in the afternoon so that you are better equipped to deal with the evening's activities.

Many people find they make better use of their time if they make lists of their immediate and long-range goals and try to devote their principal energies to the top-priority items. The complaint "I don't have time, although I'd love to do it" frequently reflects poor management and perhaps a distorted sense of values. For example, a busy mother decides that she would love to take piano lessons again, but feels she hasn't the time to practice. She tries it anyway, and suddenly finds there are a number of odd corners of time during her day where she can run a few scales.

Certainly, the basic antidote to fatigue is sleep, although chronic fatigue and lack of sleep are not necessarily related. Loss of sleep impairs judgment, slows down reaction time, and makes people jumpy and moody. Many techniques, from the humble to the scientific, have been suggested for people who have trouble getting up in the morning or falling asleep at night.

The chronic insomniac is tired because he does not sleep well. Although the immediate temptation is to reach for a bottle of sleeping pills, this habit can build into a dangerous dependency. The true insomniac would do better to consult experts at one of the many sleep laboratories around the country.

Both mild and chronic insomniacs should look at the obvious. Is the bedroom well ventilated and quiet? Sleep researchers counsel mild exercise a couple of hours before going to bed, and they caution against drinking stimulating beverages or eating heavy food just before going to bed.

For many people, exercise, whether at night or during the day, is the crucial missing element in their health picture and the one that is depriving them of a sense of well-being. First, hard physical exercise and the fatigue it produces has a tranquilizing effect on the body. Second, exercise stimulates circulation of blood to the brain, enhancing a sense of well-being. Third, exercise is a form of enjoyment, and a person who is having fun is seldom fatigued.

For busy people, getting the daily half-hour minimum of exercise which doctors prescribe may mean looking for ways of exercising that do not involve setting aside special time. The cheapest and most practical form of exercise is walking. If possible, walk to work or to the train or bus. Walk to the grocery store instead of driving. And walk upstairs instead of taking an elevator. Look for ways of moving your body.

Along with exercise, a proper diet is an essential requirement for a nonfatiguable constitution. This means knowing the basic four food categories and how much of each is required; knowing what is a sensible weight-loss diet and what is merely fatiguing and unrewarding; drinking in moderation. Various groups such as the American Heart Association, the American Medical Association, and Weight Watchers have worked out diets guaranteed to help you lose weight, maintain the loss, and eat in a healthy fashion without becoming bored or feeling put upon.

The old wisdom holds that a hearty breakfast provides an energetic start to the day. This wisdom has been called into question by some nutritionists who point out that many healthy, energetic people eat almost nothing in the morning. There is no one "ideal breakfast," and certainly anyone who is conscious of the current epidemic of heart disease in this country would feel guilty about sitting down to the classical American menu of bacon and eggs every day.

The myth of the good breakfast is not the only one which does not hold up to scientific scrutiny. Many people believe that without supplements of vitamins or energy drugs, their bodies will not function properly. Today the question of whether excess doses of vitamins do anything more than drain the pocketbook remains unanswered. Of course, the power of positive thinking cannot be discounted: The person who believes his vitamin E pills or his amino acid tablets are curing his fatigue may actually find himself less tired.

These vitamin poppers are often the same people who turn to amphetamines or barbiturates, with sometimes serious results. Tired people who believe that lack of sleep is the basis of their problem are easily led to acquire the sleeping-pill habit. While an occasional sleeping pill is helpful, extended use builds up a potentially dangerous tolerance, and it also disturbs normal sleep patterns.

Amphetamines, the "uppers" that a tired person may convince himself will solve the problem, are not physically addictive, but they can create a psychological dependency. Amphetamine abuse can lead to paranoid psychosis or accidental death. The usefulness of these drugs is limited to very specific medical situations.

The first prerequisite for freedom from fatigue, then, is a healthy body. The second prerequisite, often closely tied to the first, is a healthy mind. Doctors estimate that perhaps 80 per cent of the legions of patients who complain of fatigue are talking about an emotional and not a physical problem. To a large extent, this psychological fatigue reflects the special stresses of twentieth-century living. Many of us live in crowded urban conditions and work in high-pressure situations; unlike our rural ancestors, we cannot go out and hoe a row of beans or walk through an apple orchard when the going gets tough.

Frequently, however, the stress sufferer's condition is self-engendered, the consequence of a distorted view of life. Some people are attuned to a competitive life style which puts achievement as life's top priority; others feel that life has placed unfair burdens on them. In either case, a realistic evaluation of goals and expectations is called for.

Several researchers have pointed out that the chief sources of stress are not the conditions of modern life, but the personal disruptions to which no on is immune. Their advice: In a time of crisis, such as family breakup or economic difficulty, try to take off the pressure in other areas. For example, if your child is suffering a serious illness, do not choose that time to try to find a different job or to mortgage a new house.

Fatigue is closely bound to two frequent psychological manifestations of stress: anxiety and depression. Although for some neurotic people anxiety is a constant state which reflects a deep sense of inadequacy, normal anxiety is an inescapable part of living. Frequently it accompanies a change in a person's situation, such as a move to a distant state, and the anxiety retreats once the new situation has been accepted.

Chronically anxious people usually need the help of a professional, but they can take certain measures on their own, and without the crutches of pills or alcohol. Many anxious people suffer excessively from a sense of isolation, and their loneliness is often overcome by joining a group of some sort, whether it be consciousness raising, choral singing, or a church sewing circle. There are also specific techniques for helping a person to relax or to shake a mood.

Depression is an even more pervasive problem than anxiety, and one that is almost universally accompanied by fatigue. Today, treatment of neurotic depression consists of psychotherapy or physical therapy. The drugs available are very strong, and the mildly depressed person is better off with psychotherapy alone (shock treatments are also reserved for extreme cases).

According to Freud's widely accepted theory, depression is hostility turned inwards. In other words, the depressed person cannot afford to allow himself to drown in his feelings, but must come to terms with problems lying beneath the surface. While friends and relatives can provide moral support, long-range hope for the neurotically depressed person rests on professional assistance.

The depression brought on by circumstances, such as death or failure, is not neurotic, and will generally disappear within six months. Yet even when depression is based in reality, psychiatric counseling can be of help, particularly when the sufferer has few "willing ears" to whom he can turn.

While treatment of anxiety and depression can be lengthy and costly, there is one cause of fatigue that lends itself quite easily to self-help: boredom. Innumerable cases of fatigue are built on a chronically bored attitude toward life. This is particularly true for "tired housewives"—educated women who are at home raising a family and who find themselves having to answer to many demands, yet none of them stimulating.

Human beings start to go to pieces in an environment bereft of stimulation, as many experiments have proved. If a person is mired in a life pattern where nothing changes and where each day is predictable, he may become bored and tired.

The first line of attack: Is it possible to make a major change? Could the tired housewife hire a housekeeper and start going to law school? Could the weary breadwinner change jobs or move to a different part of the country?

Frequently, dramatic change is not possible, although the idea should at least be considered. Perhaps the feeling that "it's out of the question" is based not on circumstances, but on a timidity and fear of change. Think about it: What have you got to lose?

If extreme moves are not possible, consider alternatives that are within reach. We have all heard the advice to "find a new interest," and the fact is that once you open your life to wider horizons, you have a much better chance of not being bored.

Many people are bored because they feel useless to themselves and to others. For them, a service project may be the solution. The local YMCA, YMHA, church groups, and other community groups are always in need of help, and it is not necessary to have a particular "skill." Often the main talent sought is the ability to work patiently with people.

Others are bored because they have ceased to use their minds for anything more complex than figuring out the monthly budget. If you feel that your brain is drying up, hark back to your school days: What classes roused your interest? Perhaps you were good at languages: Why not learn the language of the largest ethnic population in your area and try to get involved in projects with them?

Many suggestions for getting a new slant on life have been offered in the pages of this book: Each person must figure out what works best for him. Generally, the prescription for fighting boredom is the prescription for fighting almost any kind of emotional fatigue: Try to develop your inner resources—imagination, perception, contemplation—rather than looking always in the exterior world for satisfactions. Open the windows of your mind.